SIMWARS SIMULATION CASE BOOK:
EMERGENCY MEDICINE

SIMWARS SIMULATION CASE BOOK: EMERGENCY MEDICINE

Edited by

LISA JACOBSON, MD

University of Florida College of Medicine, Jacksonville, FL, USA

YASUHARU OKUDA, MD

University of Central Florida College of Medicine and Veterans Health Administration, Jacksonville, FL, USA

STEVEN A. GODWIN, MD

University of Florida College of Medicine, Jacksonville, FL, USA

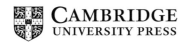

CAMBRIDGE
UNIVERSITY PRESS

University Printing House, Cambridge CB2 8BS, United Kingdom

Cambridge University Press is part of the University of Cambridge.

It furthers the University's mission by disseminating knowledge in the pursuit of
education, learning and research at the highest international levels of excellence.

www.cambridge.org
Information on this title: www.cambridge.org/9781107625280

First published 2015

Printed in the United Kingdom by Bell and Bain Ltd

A catalogue record for this publication is available from the British Library

Library of Congress Cataloguing in Publication data
SimWars simulation case book : emergency medicine / edited by Lisa Jacobson, Yasuharu
Okuda, Steven Godwin.
        p. ; cm.
Includes bibliographical references and index.
ISBN 978-1-107-62528-0 (Paperback)
I. Jacobson, Lisa (Physician), editor.   II. Okuda, Yasuharu, editor.   III. Godwin, Steven,
editor. [DNLM: 1. Emergencies–Case Reports.   2. Competency-Based Education–
Case Reports.   3. Diagnosis, Differential–Case Reports.   4. Emergency Medicine–
methods–Case Reports.   5. Patient Simulation–Case Reports. WB 105]
RA975.5.E5
362.18–dc23   2014027837

ISBN 978-1-107-62528-0 Paperback

Contents

Appendix B and Appendix C images are also available at
www.cambridge.org/9781107625280

Contributors

Neal Aaron, DO
Department of Emergency Medicine, University of Florida, Jacksonville, FL, USA

Yuemi An-Grogan, MD
Department of Emergency Medicine, Northwestern University, Chicago, IL, USA

Brian Bausano, MD
Department of Emergency Medicine, University of Missouri, Columbia, MO, USA

Michael Cassara, MD
Department of Emergency Medicine, Hofstra North Shore-LIJ School of Medicine, Manhasset, NY, USA

Becky Damazo, PNP, MSN
Rural Northern California Clinical Simulation Center, Chico, CA, USA

Michael Falk, MD
Department of Emergency Medicine, Mount Sinai St. Luke's/Roosevelt Hospital, New York, USA

Jeremy Samuel Faust, MD, MS, MA
Mount Sinai Hospital Department of Emergency Medicine, New York and Elmhurst Hospital Center, Queens, NY, USA

Aaron Gingrich, MD
Emergency Department, Bronx Lebanon Hospital Center, Bronx, NY, USA

Brandon J. Godbout, MD
Department of Emergency Medicine, Lenox Hill Hospital, North Shore – Long Island Jewish Health System, New York, USA

Steven A. Godwin, MD
Department of Emergency Medicine, University of Florida, College of Medicine, Jacksonville, FL, USA

Scott Goldberg, MD, MPH
Division of Emergency Medicine, Brigham and Women's Hospital, Boston, MA, USA

Kelvin Harold, MD
Department of Emergency Medicine, University of Florida College of Medicine, Jacksonville, FL, USA

Jessica Hernandez, MD
Emergency Medicine Simulation Education, Einstein Healthcare Network, Philadelphia, PA, USA

Lisa Jacobson, MD
University of Florida College of Medicine, Jacksonville, FL, USA

Jennifer Johnson, MD
Department of Emergency Medicine, St. Vincent's Medical Center, Jacksonville, FL, USA

Nikita K. Joshi, MD
Stanford University, Stanford, CA, USA

Marianne Juarez, MD
Department of Emergency Medicine, University of California at San Francisco, San Francisco, CA, USA

Jared M. Kutzin, DNP, MS, MPH, RN, CPPS
Winthrop University Hospital, Mineola, NY, USA

Kristin McKee, DO
Department of Emergency Medicine, University
of Florida College of Medicine, Jacksonville,
FL, USA

Jacqueline A. Nemer, MD, FACEP
Department of Emergency Medicine, University
of California at San Francisco, San Francisco,
CA, USA

Jeanne A. Noble, MD MA
Department of Emergency Medicine, University
of California at San Francisco, San Francisco,
CA, USA

Yasuharu Okuda, MD
University of Central Florida College of Medicine and SimLEARN, Veterans Health Administration, Jacksonville, FL, USA

Viril Patel, MD
Department of Emergency Medicine, St. Lukes/
Roosevelt Hospital, New York, NY, USA

Kevin Reed, MD
Department of Emergency Medicine, MedStar
Harbor Hospital, Baltimore, MD, USA

Nicholas Renz, MD
Department of Emergency Medicine, Washington University in St. Louis, St. Louis, MO, USA

David Salzman, MD
Department of Emergency Medicine, Northwestern University, Chicago, IL, USA

Christopher Sampson, MD
Department of Emergency Medicine, University
of Missouri, Columbia, MO, USA

Andrew Schmidt, DO, MPH
Department of Emergency Medicine, University
of Florida, Jacksonville, FL, USA

Kirill Shishlov, MD
Department of Emergency Medicine, Mount Sinai
St. Luke's/Roosevelt Hospital, New York, USA

Michael Smith, MD
Department of Emergency Medicine, Cleveland
Clinic/Metro Health, Cleveland, OH, USA

Christopher G. Strother, MD
Department of Emergency Medicine, Pediatrics,
and Education, Icahn School of Medicine at
Mount Sinai, New York, USA

Julian Villar, MD, MPH
Department of Emergency Medicine, University
of California at San Francisco, San Francisco,
CA, USA

Jason Wagner, MD
Department of Emergency Medicine, Washing-
ton University in St. Louis, St. Louis, MO,
USA

Ernest Wang, MD, FACEP
NorthShore University HealthSystem, Evanston
and Department of Emergency Medicine,
University of Chicago Pritzker School of
Medicine, Chicago, IL, USA

Scott D. Weingart, MD, FCCM
Department of Emergency Medicine, Icahn
School of Medicine, Elmhurst Hospital, New
York, USA

Preface

The experiences in this book that are re-created as patient care scenarios are a compilation of multiple patient encounters over our careers. Our hope and great desire is that through the use of this material providers will be able to enhance their methods to provide more creative and effective training, with the ultimate goal of helping patients and impacting overall patient care outcomes.

We are grateful for the privilege of sharing this knowledge and these experiences with the reader and appreciate the wonderful support that we have received from family and colleagues as this material was developed.

Abbreviations and units

ABBREVIATIONS

ABCDE	airway, breathing, circulation, disability and exposure
ABG	arterial blood gases
AC	accessory cephalic vein
ACLS	advanced cardiovascular life support
ACS	acute coronary syndrome
AND	allow natural death
ALP	alkaline phosphatase (U/L)
ALT	alanine aminotransferase (U/L)
AST	aspartate aminotransferase (U/L)
BiPAP	bilevel positive airway pressure
BLS	basic life support
BMP	basic metabolic panel
BP	blood pressure (mmHg)
BS	breath sounds
BUN	blood urea nitrogen (mg/dL)
BVM	bag valve mask
CBC	complete blood count
CHF	congestive heart failure
CPK	creatine phosphokinase
CPR	Cardiopulmonary resuscitation
CTA	clear to ausculation
CTAB	clear to ausculation bilaterally
CVA	cerebrovascular accident
CXR	chest radiograph
DNR	do not resuscitate
DOA	drugs of abuse
ED	emergency department
EEG	electroencephalography
EKG	electrocardiography
EMS	emergency medical services/personnel
ESR	erythrocyte sedimentation rate
ETCO$_2$	end-tidal carbon dioxide

ETT	endotracheal tube
FAST	focused assessment with sonography in trauma
FiO_2	fraction of inspired oxygen
GCS	Glasgow Coma Scale
GI	gastrointestinal
HEENT	head, eyes, ears, nose and throat examination
Hgb	hemoglobin (g/dL)
HPI	history of presenting illness
HR	heart rate (beats/min)
ICP	intracranial pressure
ICU	intensive care unit
IM	intramuscular
INR	international normalized ratio
IO	intraosseous access
IV	intravenous
IVC	inferior vena cava
JVD	jugular vein distention
LFT	liver function test
LP	lumbar puncture
LT	laryngeal tube
MAP	mean arterial pressure (mmHg)
MI	myocardial infarction
MICU	medical intensive care unit
m/r/g	murmurs/rubs/gallops
NC	nasal cannula
NG	nasogastric
NICU	neonatal intensive care unit
NKDA	no known drug allergies
NRB	non-rebreather mask
O_2 Sat	oxygen saturation (%)
OR	operating room
PALS	pediatric advanced life support
PCO_2	partial pressure carbon dioxide (mmHg)
PEA	pulseless electrical activity
PEEP	positive end-expiratory pressure
PEERL	pupils equal, round, reactive to light
PICU	pediatric intensive care unit
PMD	primary medical doctor
PMH	past medical history
PO_2	partial pressure oxygen (mmHg)
PRBC	peripheral red blood cells
PT	prothrombin time
PTT	partial thromboplastin time
RA	room air
ROSC	return of spontaneous circulation
RR	respiratory rate (breaths/min)
RSI	rapid sequence intubation
SC	subcutaneous

TPA	tissue plasminogen activator
US	ultrasound
VBG	venous blood gases
VS	vital signs
WBC	white blood cell count
XR	radiograph

UNITS

	Unit	Reference range/normal
Bicarbonate	mEq/L	22–28
BUN	mg/dL	8–18
Calcium	mg/dL (mmol/L)	8.5–10.2 (2.25–2.5)
Chloride	mEq/L	95–105
Creatinine	mg/dL	0.6–1.2
Glucose	mg/dL	70–110
Hematocrit	%	33–43 (female), 39–49 (male)
Hemoglobin	g/dL	12–15(female), 12.6–17.2 (male)
Lactate	mmol/L	1.0–1.8
Liver enzymes	U/L	AST 5–40, ALT 7–56, ALP 30–120)
$PaCO_2$	mmHg	40
PaO_2	mmHg	100 (FiO_2 0.21)
pH		7.35–7.45
Platelets	$\times\ 10^3/mm^3$	150–450
Potassium	mEq/L	3.5–5
O_2 Sats (FiO_2 0.21)	%	97–100
Sodium	mEq/L	135–145
White blood cell count	$\times\ 10^3/mm^3$	3.2–9.8

PART I

SIMWARS 101

CHAPTER 1

Why SimWars?

Steven A. Godwin

BACKGROUND

Why SimWars is an interesting question that requires some background to fully understand the driving forces behind the educational program's development. As simulation training has evolved, concurrent increased utilization across specialties has also occurred. Leaders in the field of simulation developed courses centered around crisis resource management based on communication and safety principles. In parallel, in many medical schools, a changing paradigm of medical education that focuses less on large-group didactics and more on small-group interaction has also emerged. Likewise, learners have come to expect more innovative approaches to educational conferences. Unique training experiences can, therefore, be very important when engaging resident learners.

A study conducted in 2008 showed that 85% of emergency residency programs use mannequin-based simulation in the training of their residents. The Accreditation Council for Graduate Medical Education (ACGME) now requires internal medicine residency programs to "provide residents with access to training using simulation" and accepts simulation to access competency in up to 30% of required procedures for emergency medicine.

Unfortunately the same 2008 study illustrated that faculty time constraints and lack of trained faculty (66% and 54%, respectively) were the main barriers to simulation use in their programs. Unlike the traditional model of graduate medical training, using lecture format to teach large groups of learners, the challenge to simulation-based education is that it requires faculties to have expertise in simulation case development, facilitation and debriefing. It also often requires a significant amount of faculty time and resources, as sessions are often facilitated in a small 1 to 4 trainer to learner ratio, in order to create realism and maintain a safe learning environment.

NEEDS ASSESSMENT

Medicine in general, and particularly emergency medicine, is a team sport but for much of our history the focus on learning has been on individual performance. Certainly individual performance in a clinical environment is key to ensuring good patient care, but it alone is not enough to provide the best care possible to the patient and their families. Clearly medicine has been slower than many fields, such as the military, aviation and industry, in recognizing the importance of team training for optimal performance. As team training and crisis resource management began to be formulated from specialties such as anesthesia, use of simulation training emerged as an innovative and effective method to train team performance. Emergency medicine also appeared as a natural area for its application. Safety projects like MedTeams emerged that increased awareness for this type of performance standards. However, the issues regarding available time and expertise of instructors beg at least two questions: "Where is there time to add team training and ultimately patient safety concepts into already packed training curricula and conference agendas?" and "How could one increase participation and expand awareness of these concepts while creating an entertaining learning environment?".

Clinical pathology case conferences have provided educational theater for medical conferences while challenging individuals and also creating a sense of departmental accomplishment and pride. Could a similar event be created that harnessed that same competitive academic spirit in a simulated format? As this concept was being considered, a popular television program, *American Idol*, highlighted a singing competition with immediate feedback from judges to the performers. This focused and directed feedback is given not only to the participants but also to the audience. Interestingly, it was recognized that this immediate feedback had the potential to reflect what is commonly done with bedside teaching in an instructor–learner encounter. Unlike the show where feedback was neither constructive nor often professional, what if the entertaining qualities of the feedback could be adopted while still maintaining professional respect for the learner and the participants? Such feedback, in simulated encounters with limited time spans, would clearly not be able to completely follow well accepted and studied debriefing strategies; however, some tools could certainly transfer over, for example simple delta strategies for; discovery.

What would make individuals want to participate in front of their peers at risk of embarrassment and potential shame if giving a poor performance? What makes us compete in athletic events where others may observe or be aware of the outcome? The privilege and challenge of being able to care for patients' lives far exceeds the stakes of athletic events. Having the opportunity to challenge oneself in a team-based patient encounter provides an opportunity to observe professional performance in lifelike circumstances. The desire to compete on behalf of one's home training program and institution becomes a driving force that encourages the normally less extroverted individual to willingly perform with colleagues in front of their peers.

A main goal in the development of SimWars was to create a learning experience that in some manner addressed each of the highlighted questions. SimWars' competitions provide the challenge of a clinical dilemma that unfolds over brief 8 minute encounters in a competitive environment. The structure allows the audience to mentally participate with the learners as they are actively performing the scenario. After completion of each scenario, the audience actually becomes the learner as the expert panel discusses key learning objectives encountered during the case. In addition to the clinical knowledge, procedural and communication skills that are highlighted, simulation training techniques and strategies are also demonstrated. This mix of training objectives allows the event to meet the mission of not only providing clinical education but also of expanding simulation training. Audiences and participants leave the competition with a broad working experience in both simple and complex simulation training techniques that can be taken back to their home institutions.

Ultimately, SimWars fills the need of providing small-group education to large-group audiences. Audiences are active participants as they vote for the winner of each case competition. As observers critique the competing teams, a greater sense of engagement is created, as they become active members of the educational process.

Why SimWars? The answer may vary for the purpose of the conference itself but the driving principle is to provide a unique and challenging learning experience that engages both the participants and the observers.

BIBLIOGRAPHY

Howard SK, Gaba DM, Fish KJ et al. Anesthesia crisis resource management training: teaching anesthesiologists to handle critical incidents. *Aviat Space Environ Med* 1992; 63:763–770.
Okuda Y, Bond W, Bonfante G et al. National growth in simulation training within emergency medicine residency programs, 2003–2008. *Acad Emerg Med* 2008; 15(11):1113–1116.

CHAPTER 2

What is SimWars

Yasuharu Okuda

The use of mannequin-based simulation to train healthcare providers has evolved significantly over the decades. Initially championed by experts such as David Gaba to develop highly effective clinical teams using crisis management principles derived from the aviation industry, simulation has now become a staple training tool for healthcare training programs.

The authors of this book created a training competition, entitled SimWars, to maximize the value of simulation across a large group of learners while maintaining the benefits seen in facilitated small group simulation encounters. SimWars also increases the ability for clinical experts and other non-simulation faculty members to increase participation in simulation-based training without having to become experts in simulation. This book defines the SimWars program, describes how to implement SimWars in a department, hospital or organization and provides over 40 emergency medicine cases previously vetted at national SimWars competitions. Each of the cases is linked to the ACGME milestones.

SimWars is a simulation-based clinical competition where teams of residents or clinical providers come together to compete against one another on simulated patient scenarios in front of a live audience. Upon completion of each case, a panel of judges, selected on their clinical background and simulation-based training expertise, provides debriefing feedback to the team members based on the team's clinical management, procedural skills, teamwork and communication. The audience votes on the team with the best performance, and the winning teams progress through the competition in a single-elimination tournament format until there is only one team left standing.

SimWars was created by Yasuharu Okuda, Andy Godwin and Scott Weingart in 2007 and first implemented during the New York City Emergency Department Critical Care Conference held at the Icahn School of Medicine at Mount Sinai. Initially started with minimal resources and staff, SimWars has now evolved into collaborative effort between individuals, academic organizations, and vendors. Since its inception, it has now been held around the world in over 30 national and international meetings including of the American College of Emergency Physicians and the Society for Academic Emergency Medicine and the International Meeting on Simulation in Healthcare. The competition has also evolved into other disciplines including meetings in oral maxillofacial surgery, gynecology, and neurocritical care, and to countries from Canada to Australia.

For emergency medicine, Lisa Jacobson was named the first national director responsible for program management and senior editor for the SimWars cases. Funding was obtained through grants and other resources provided by the Emergency Medicine Residents Association and the Foundation for Education and Research for Neurologic Emergencies. Case development and other staff support were provided by the Society for Academic Emergency Medicine's Simulation Academy.

THE FORMAT

The SimWars competition is held in a single-elimination format with two teams (A and B) competing against one another on the same simulation scenario (Fig. 2.1), with the order decided by a coin toss. The team performing second is asked to leave the room, to blind them to the scenario and its respective management by the first team. Upon completion of the scenario, a panel of three expert judges debriefs the first team's members on their performance. When the first team is done being debriefed, the second team is then invited back into the room to go through the same scenario, which is again debriefed by the judges. At this point, the moderator asks the audience to vote on the winner based on what they observed and judges' input, using an audience response system. Depending on the total number of teams, this format is repeated using new cases until there is only one SimWars champion team. The sample format (Fig. 2.1) and schedule (Table 2.1) are shown for a competition involving four teams, with team C as the winner in this example.

The teams

Teams typically have four members. For emergency medicine residency competitions, a minimum of one senior resident is required with the remaining three members composed of any combination of postgraduate levels.

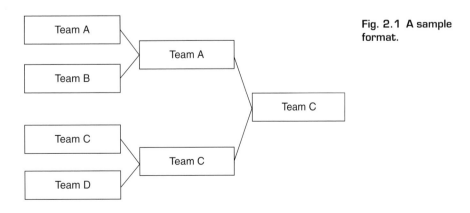

Fig. 2.1 A sample format.

TABLE 2.1 SAMPLE SCHEDULE

	Time	Case	Event
Round 1	7:00–7:10		Introduction
Team A vs. B	7:10–7:20	1	Team A
	7:20–7:30		Debrief
	7:30–7:40	1	Team B
	7:40–7:50		Debrief
Team C vs. D	7:50–8:00	2	Team C
	8:00–8:10		Debrief
	8:10–8:20	2	Team D
	8:20–8:30		Debrief
Finals	8:30–8:40	3	Team A
	8:40–8:50		Debrief
	8:50–9:00	3	Team C (winner)
	9:00–9:10		Debrief

The moderator

Moderators have an extremely important function. Besides facilitation and maintaining the schedule of the competition, their job is to set clear expectations from the beginning for the teams, judges and audience members. Below are some speaking points during the introduction.

- For the teams
  - the purpose of the SimWars Competition is to have a friendly inter-residency competition, focused on learning
  - we will try to maintain as safe a learning environment as possible but realize that SimWars is still a competition. There is a clear winner at the end
  - you will be judged equally on teamwork, communication and clinical management
  - use of any reference or mobile device is allowed if these are typically used during your clinical shift
  - if you are unclear about a finding, ask the confederate (actor) nurse.
- For the judges
  - we expect the judges to be professional but be honest with feedback, both positive and negative
  - disagreement is healthy and is encouraged amongst the judges
  - judges will be responsible for selecting a winner on the final round only
  - judges will have 10 minutes total to give feedback to each team.
- For the audience
  - will be voting on the winner of each round, except the final round, based on the judges' input and your observation of the team's performance
  - we expect you to vote based on merit and not popularity
  - only one vote per audience member is allowed.

At this point, the teams are introduced and the schedule is announced. Each team has 10 minutes per case.

The other role of the moderator is to maintain a fun atmosphere, to keep the competition light hearted. If a particular judge appears to be too harsh or if the moderator notices a team member is upset, it is up to the moderator to step in to smooth things out. Typically this can be accomplished by refocusing the group on the main purpose of SimWars, which is to learn about clinical management and teamwork skills in a fun competitive environment. Other techniques include recognizing the participant's willingness to compete in front of a live audience for the sake of learning and their residency program.

The judges

Proper judge selection is critical to the success of the SimWars competition. The key is to have a balanced panel of three judges with a mix of clinical subject matter, simulation learning background and debriefing, and teamwork and communication expertise. In addition, the judges should have strong personalities, which makes the discussion fun, entertaining and safe. For further information on judging, please refer to Chapters 4 and 5.

THE CASES

SimWars competitions at previously held emergency medicine meetings have been based on clinical themes such as "altered mental status," "toxicology" and "environmental emergencies." The purpose of choosing a theme is to focus the learning on a topic, increase the ease of recruiting the appropriate judge(s) and reduce case repetition over time.

Once the theme is selected, case ideas are brainstormed with a small group of simulation and clinical content experts. Given the short 8–10 minute time frame, proper case selection is key to a successful SimWars event. If the case is too simple, the team will be done too quickly. If the case is too complicated, with an excessive number of goals and objectives, the team will either stray off track or complete only a part of the scenario before time is over. The ideal case has two to three main clinical decision points, overlaid with a couple of distractors, and one or two communication or teamwork challenges. Some examples are given.

Too simple

A 64-year-old woman with chest pain radiating to the left arm, associated with nausea and diaphoresis. States pain feels like an elephant is sitting on her chest. No associate symptoms. No allergies. No medications. Family history of MI. EKG shows anterior wall ST elevations with reciprocal changes. The patient is in the ED during the daytime, and the cardiac catheterization lab is available.

- Diagnosis and management of anterior STEMI (clinical)
- Communication with cardiologist (communication)
- (no distractor).

Too complicated
A 64-year-old Chinese-speaking (minimal English) woman with chest pain radiating to the left arm and back, associated with shortness of breath, nausea and diaphoresis. Unable to describe character of chest pain. Unable to elicit other symptoms. Accompanied by husband who is drunk and combative. Patient is allergic to aspirin and takes multiple herbal medications. Physical exam shows multiple bruises over body of varying ages and patient tearful. EKG shows anterior wall ST elevations with reciprocal changes. D-dimer elevated. The patient is in the ED at night, in a small community hospital with no night-time cardiology availability. Unable to get interpreter.

- Differential diagnosis of chest pain (clinical)
  - ▶ cardiac (clinical)
  - ▶ dissection (clinical)
  - ▶ pulmonary embolism (clinical)
- Aspirin allergy in possible acute coronary syndrome (ACS) (clinical)
- Alternative medicine/herbal remedies associated with chest pain (clinical)
- Transfer issues (clinical)
- Consent issues (communication)
- Communication with patient, obtaining an interpreter (communication)
- Spousal abuse (clinical/social)
- Disruptive behaviors (distractor).

Just right
A 64-year-old Chinese-speaking (minimal English) woman with chest pain radiating to the left arm, associated with shortness of breath, nausea and diaphoresis. States pain feels like an elephant is sitting on her chest. No associate symptoms. Accompanied by husband who is bilingual and can translate. Patient has no known drug allergies and takes multiple herbal medications. EKG shows anterior wall ST elevations with reciprocal changes. The patient is in the ED at night, in a small community hospital with no night-time cardiology availability. Unable to get an official interpreter. Wife and husband do not believe in Western medicine and do not want any IV medications but want pain to stop.

- Diagnosis and management of anterior STEMI (clinical)
- Transfer patient for cardiac catheterization vs. thrombolysis (clinical)
- Alternative medicine/herbal remedies associated with chest pain (clinical)
- Obtaining consent vs. refusal to be treated (communication/distractor)
- Issues with using family as the interpreter (communication)
- Wants pain to stop (distractor).

The winner

The audience votes for the winner of each round, based on observation and judges' feedback, until the final round. The winner of the final round is decided by the judges to ensure merit-based selection over popularity. Each member of the winning team and residency program receives a plaque and is automatically invited back the following year as returning champions to defend their title as SimWars champions.

SUMMARY

SimWars has now entered its eighth year with demand rapidly growing outside of emergency medicine. The popularity of SimWars stems from its unique blend of bedside teaching, entertainment and simulation-based competition. It allows clinical content experts, without simulation expertise, to participate as judges, while expanding simulation-based learning to a larger audience. SimWars also offers multiple opportunities for faculty development and scholarship, which includes scenario case writer, facilitation and judging. As simulation continues to become an integral part of interdisciplinary and medical specialty training, there is a growing need for simulation-based training resources. The following cases include many of the previously vetted emergency medicine SimWars cases and include teaching points and visual stimuli to allow the reader to easily reproduce our library of high-quality simulation-based teaching cases.

BIBLIOGRAPHY

Dong C, Clapper T, Szyld D. A qualitative descriptive study of SimWars as a meaningful instructional tool. *Int J Med Educ* 2013; 3:139–145.

Fehr JJ, Honkanen A, Murray D. Simulation in pediatric anesthesiology. *Pediatr Anesth* 2012; 22:988–994.

Howard SK, Gaba DM, Fish KJ et al. Anesthesia crisis resource management training: teaching anesthesiologists to handle critical incidents. *Aviat Space Environ Med* 1992; 63:763–770.

McLaughlin S, Clarke S, Menon S et al. Simulation in emergency medicine. In Leving A, DeMaria S, et al. eds., *The Comprehensive Textbook of Healthcare Simulation*. New York: Springer, 2013, pp. 315–328.

Okuda Y, Bond W, Bonfante G et al. National growth in simulation training within emergency medicine residency programs, 2003–2008. *Acad Emerg Med* 2008; 15(11):1113–1116.

Okuda Y, Godwin A, Westenbarger R et al. "Sim Wars" a new edge to academic residency competitions. *Acad Emerg Med* 2009; 16:S326–S376.

SimHealth2011 at the *Annual Conference of the Australian Society for Simulation Healthcare* (http://www.simulationaustralia.org.au/archive/simtect/2011SH/gallery/650.html, accessed 30 July 2014).

SIMTREK, the Royal College of Physicians and Surgeons of Canada 2014 competition (http://www.royalcollege.ca/portal/page/portal/rc/events/simulationsummit/simwars, accessed 30 July 2014).

CHAPTER 3

SimWars: how to succeed

Lisa Jacobson

Chapters 1 and 2 outlined some of the what and why of SimWars. This chapter describes more about how to make SimWars happen at your next conference.

WHO?

Who makes up the creative team, the production team, the competing teams? The following is typical:

- teams
  - typically have three to four members
  - should have similar make-ups (e.g. all residents, two physicians and two nurses, etc.)
  - should be recruited in advance
- judges/expert panel: see the other chapters for more information
- audience: vote via audience response system for the winning team in all rounds except the finals
- confederates
  - students, residents, simulation technicians, educators and volunteer actors can all be confederates
  - require intimate knowledge of the case to facilitate its flow
  - provide information necessary to make the case progress, typically as nurse observations, consultants, EMS hand-offs, family members with history
  - control the flow of time by performing actual patient care activities or withholding information
  - often serve as distracters/confounders providing challenges in the case as well as entertainment
- facilitator
  - has ultimate control of flow and time
  - cues confederates and simulation wizard
  - releases results (labs, images), typically in the form of a power point slide show
  - adapts to unexpected occurrences in the simulation

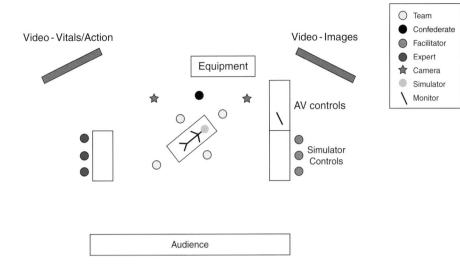

Fig. 3.1 A possible room layout.

■ simulation wizard
  ▶ works the simulator, which is run "on the fly" to accommodate unexpected participant decisions
  ▶ may be the voice of the simulator.

WHERE?

Where do all of these moving pieces go? Layout is given in Fig. 3.1.

■ If possible, set up in an auditorium with a stage.
■ Project the action, and the important clinical information (vital signs, images) on screens adjacent to the stage.
■ Set up center stage as a clinical environment, with supplies, the mannequin and room for the managing team as well as the confederates.
■ Set up tables to one side for the judges and at another one for the technical support.
■ If the action moves off stage, have the camera vantage follow it.

HOW

It is helpful to see a SimWars before attempting to create one. A combination of creativity, spontaneity and logistical oversight is necessary for success. The model that has become successful will be briefly described below with the layout shown in Fig. 3.1.

1. Start planning early. This includes submitting a course proposal to the conference of choice (see the sample proposal below).
2. Work with a team. The list to coordinate includes (but is not limited to):
   ▶ room reservation and layout
   ▶ AV equipment: video integration, microphones for competitors and confederates
   ▶ mannequin confirmation
   ▶ medical equipment
   ▶ team recruitment
   ▶ judge recruitment

▶ confederate recruitment
▶ case creation
▶ moulage.

3. Create challenging cases with simple flow:
   ▶ choose a theme
   ▶ focus on critical teaching points
   ▶ make sure cases are reproducible
   ▶ add confounders to distract, entertain and create realism.

4. Connect each case with necessary moulage and confederates to produce fidelity. This may include sounds, smells, visual stimuli and more.

5. Run through the cases with your confederates before the actual event: their knowledge of the case flow will help to facilitate the release of information to the competitors.

6. During the introduction, be sure to clarify some important components of SimWars:
   ▶ this is not safe learning
   ▶ the audience will vote in all rounds but the finals for the advancing team
   ▶ the judges will choose the ultimate winner.

7. Divide responsibility. If possible, different members of your leadership team should have different roles on the day of the competition:
   ▶ SimWizard should manage the mannequin in real time
   ▶ the facilitator should manage the flow of the case and may also control the power point of visual stimuli.

8. AV resources need to be controlled:
   ▶ audio control of microphone power, volume and interference
   ▶ visual control of camera angles, split the screen, record for posterity.

TIPS

■ Set the ground rules for competitors in advance
   ▶ this is not safe learning
   ▶ remember to suspend disbelief.
■ Set the ground rules for judges in advance
   ▶ honest but respectful feedback helpful for audience as well as personal learning
   ▶ division of labor to include one person focused specifically on emphasizing clinical learning points helps to ensure that these points are consistently emphasized.
■ Choose a theme for the cases to focus the learning points.
■ Be prepared, but flexible – sometimes technology does not work the way you want it to.

SAMPLE PROPOSAL SUBMISSION

1. Course objectives:
   ▶ highlight critical decision making in a high stakes environment
   ▶ demonstrate effective debriefing tools in time-limited environments
   ▶ entertain and educate the audience.

2. Course co-directors:
   - ▶ Joe Smith, MD, FACEP, Director, Simulation Lab, University of Excellent Learning, USA
   - ▶ Maria Ramos, MD, FACEP, Assistant Dean, Simulation Education, University of Even Better Learning, Canada.
3. Brief course description. SimWars is an interactive simulation competition that allows teams of medical providers to compete against each other on simulated patient encounters in front of a large audience. An expert panel judges the performance of each teams in areas such as teamwork, communication and leadership as well as in the medical management of the "patient." The audience will vote on the winner of each case using the audience response system based on their direct observation and the panel's input. Each encounter will be recorded by an advanced AV system that can capture multiple views of the simulation and merge with the physiological input. Ultimately there can be only one "fill in your conference name and year" SimWars Champion.

CHAPTER 4

SimWars debriefing: the art of the show

Ernest Wang

Effective SimWars debriefing poses special challenges. SimWars is unlike traditional medical simulation training in many respects and these differences require a modified approach to debriefing so that the experience can be a memorable one.

The skillful SimWars debriefer must be able to *critique* effectively and *entertain* simultaneously. This chapter will review the features of a SimWars debriefing, the similarities and differences between SimWars and traditional simulation debriefing, and strategies for judges to most effectively conduct debriefings at SimWars events.

JUDGING SIMWARS

The SimWars judging panel typically consists of three healthcare professionals. They can be physicians, nurses, educational specialists (PhD, masters, etc.), or other allied health professionals (e.g. paramedics, respiratory therapists) depending on the specialties and composition of the teams. Historically, judges are selected because they have recognized content expertise in clinical medicine, in simulation-based education/debriefing, or both.

The judges' task is to watch teams manage a simulation case and provide commentary on the performance. Each team is judged on three areas: clinical management, teamwork and communication. Typically, the panel will decide beforehand who will critique each area. Since SimWars cases are often chaotic and loud, this allows the judges to be able to better focus on their specific element and make specific evaluations.

Each judge provides a brief analysis of their observation of the team's performance in order to help the audience to decide on a winner for the round. Additionally, the judges will provide insight into the clinical management and highlight the key teaching points of the case.

In the elimination rounds, the audience decides which of the competing teams will advance to the next round. The judges' commentaries are critical to the global evaluation of the teams' performances and provide the audience with opinions to supplement their own observations when making their choice of the winner of each round. In the championship round, in addition to providing commentary, the judges will select the overall winner.

TABLE 4.1 COMPARISION OF SIMWARS DEBRIEFING
AND TRADITIONAL DEBRIEFING

Similarities	Differences
Gather information	Competition
Analyze	"A Show"
Diagnostic feedback	Time compression
Supportive	Less time for self-reflection
Summarize	Case complexity (usually more so
Review case goals and objectives	because of competition)
Review take home points	Noise
Provide action plan	Big audience

SIMILARITIES AND DIFFERENCES TO TRADITIONAL SIMULATION DEBRIEFING

There are many similarities and differences when comparing SimWars debriefing to traditional debriefing. Some of these elements are summarized in Table 4.1.

Similarities

According to Fanning and Gaba, all simulation debriefing models utilize reflection around an experience (the scenario), discussion of the experience and the promotion of learning and behavior modification based on the reflective exercise of the debrief.

A good SimWars debrief is similar to other models in that it should allow discussion of individual and team-level performances, the identification of any errors made and development of a plan for improving a further performance.

SimWars debriefing contains many of the same elements as traditional debriefing. After each scenario, the judges structure the discussion around case management with attention to the learning objectives and team performance. The judges also provide an assessment of the performance.

Differences

SimWars is first and foremost a competition. Each round, one team will win and one team must lose. In this vein, the traditional "safe learning environment" is less applicable. Furthermore, the teams are "exposed" from the start – they are performing in front of a large public audience armed with audience response clickers.

The judging panel must be able to debrief in such a way as to make an effective argument for why one team performed better in each round. This is particularly necessary when performance of the two teams is very close. Pointing out poor or weak performances in a public forum differentiates the SimWars debriefing from the traditional simulation debrief. At times, this can be uncomfortable for the participants and/or the debriefer, particularly if there is controversy over treatment or if the management errors were significant.

Another significant difference is time constraint. Traditional debriefing theory recommends a debriefing length equal to or greater than the length of the session.

Some debriefing experts recommend no less than 30 minutes per debrief. This is clearly not feasible during a bracket-type competition.

The SimWars debrief must be completed within about 10 minutes. There is less time to explore issues and nuances or to allow for self-reflection. Diagnostic statements of performance are used in place of a traditional "advocacy-inquiry" approach, for example: "It seemed that securing the airway was difficult in this case. It would have been easier to perform had it been done at the outset before the patient developed significant angioedema."

BREAKING THE ICE

One of the most important aspects of SimWars debriefing is how the initial judge opens the discussion. For many of the teams, this experience might be the first time they have ever had to do something so stressful in front of a large audience.

Team members of a case gone bad often know right away. This can be seen in their body language and in their demeanor. They can potentially feel demoralized or humiliated.

An astute judge can quickly determine how a team feels about their performance immediately after the case. How the first judge opens the debriefing is critical and can mean the difference between a team leaving with a thoroughly bad experience or an insight-building one.

Acknowledging the difficulty of the case is a good way to break the ice. "How do you think you did?" is often not the best way to begin the debriefing when the team performed poorly. They *know* they did not manage the case well and now they have to publically admit it. Better to support them and let them know that the case was difficult and demanding; for example

> This was a rare, life-threatening case that would be difficult for anyone to manage under normal circumstances, let alone in front of a large audience...

> The management issues in this case were complex and the distractions were very disruptive.

Another tactic is to pick out who you think will be able to provide the best insights based on your viewing of the case management. Sometimes it will not be the team leader, but the team member who has observed the most.

A non-judgmental opening can help the participants to ease into the debriefing, for example

> Now that you've had a moment to collect your thoughts, <pick someone> can you tell us what the diagnosis of this case was and how you arrived at that?

After the introduction, the judges can then delve into the analysis of the case management, either with diagnostic statements of performance, or analytic questions such as

> What do you think were the critical actions in this case?

> Why do you think you had difficulty with _____ (i.e. the intubation, the hypotension, etc.)?

> If you were to redo this case now, what would you do differently?

If the team performed extremely, well, *emphasize* what they did well, commend them and provide positive reinforcement so that they will continue to do it in the later rounds.

THE ART OF THE SHOW

Polonius, in Shakespeare's *Hamlet*, says "Brevity is the soul of wit."

The "entertainment value" of SimWars is another key element in the success of the format. The cases are theatrical and complex – often involving multiple patients, many more confederates and a wide array of distractions to try and derail the teams from being able to manage the cases.

There is no question that a key element to a good SimWars debrief is the ability of the judging panel to powerfully and succinctly point out where the teams and individuals shined or faltered. Nothing kills a debrief more than a judge who provides a long, drawn-out, choppy, boring monologue that dilutes the essence of the performance: "All the world's a stage, And all the men and women merely players" (Jaques in Shakespeare's *As You Like it*).

An extremely useful exercise, if you wish to observe this type of concise, *and diagnostic* debriefing, is to watch episodes of the competitive formats such as "Dancing with the Stars," "American Idol," or "America's Got Talent." The judges have a polished approach, deliver great one-liners that summarize the performance and always convey what the particpants have to improve on if they want to make it to the next round. The popularity of these shows, in part, rely on the ability of the judges to entertain. And the feedback is generally *effective*, as the participants must incorporate the judges' feedback if they are to continue on the competition. The skillful SimWars judge must be able to interject a dose of his/her personality into the discussion.

Eye on the prize: effective strategies for SimWars judges

Having had the opportunity to judge since the inaugural event in 2008, I have found the following strategies to be very helpful in crafting a SimWars debrief.

- Concentrate on first impressions, which are critical. How you open the debriefing sets the tone for the rest of the session. This is particularly important when critiquing a poor performance. Prepare and rehearse an opening based on the case and plan for how you would debrief a successful team versus a team that struggled.
- Keep the debrief diagnostic and succinct – think "Dancing with the Stars;" for example: "I liked how your team was able to quickly and effectively establish rapport with the difficult family member. This allowed you to obtain the necessary history and manage the case successfully."
- Divide up the debrief topics among the panel members beforehand. Each judge should focus on one area primarily during each case: clinical management, teamwork or communication. This will help limit repetitive comments.
- Focus on the most decisive performance issues during the debriefing. Each case has two or three critical actions that will affect the overall clinical management. The judges must qualify how well these were performed relative to the competition. More importantly, the judges must describe how incorrect performance or omission of a critical action adversely affected the case.
- Explicitly discuss teamwork processes such as coordination, backup behavior and mutual performance monitoring. Describe specific examples of how these factors affected the teams' overall management of each case.

■ Discuss communication skills, such as active listening, two-way communication, fact finding, team talk, the use of a common language and closed-loop communication.

■ Support feedback with specifics. This can be done in a supportive way, even in a public forum. Defending the psychological safety of the participants is still important and should be promoted. This is a key skill for SimWars judges to be aware of and practice. For example: "The reason that the patient coded was because there was a delay in the recognition of ventricular fibrillation. The entire team seemed preoccupied with the airway and no one was paying attention to the monitor."

■ Leave them with goals. Provide suggestions, such as "Your team skillfully managed (tasks X, Y, and Z), but in order to be successful in the next round, you will need to improve your closed-loop communication. There were several instances where orders were shouted out but no one acknowledged them or confirmed that they were done."

■ Save self-reflection for the end if there is time.

■ Summarize the take-home points for the audience. Provide the players and the audience with the essence of each case. Did they meet the goals and objectives? If so, how well? What aspects of the performance were key to their success or defeat? Provide them with a sense of closure and make the take-home message stick.

■ Act and practice! Yes, judges have to practice too. Write down your "lines" such as in the examples above beforehand, rehearse them out loud. Be dynamic and polished in delivery. The message will be more memorable and powerful.

QUESTION FOR DEBATE

There are some who question whether SimWars promotes the type of "deep reflection" necessary for changing behavior. We have consistently observed that teams listen to the judges' assessments. They incorporate the diagnostic feedback, they tweak their team performance based on how they performed in the previous case. The competitive nature of the event amplifies the experience and the teams almost always perform significantly better in each round, with respect to teamwork and communication, in particular.

SUMMARY

Debriefing a SimWars competition requires a framework that differs from traditional simulation debriefing paradigms. The judges' job is to clearly and quickly convey what the teams *did* well, what they *did not do* well and what they *must do better* in order to advance in this competition. There is less time for self-reflection and the judges spend more time analyzing and summarizing the performance.

More importantly, a premium is placed on the ability to skillfully balance the provision of a *judgment* on their performance in a public forum while preserving participants' self-esteem in the face of positive and negative (possibly critical) diagnostic feedback.

Carried out properly, SimWars debriefing can be efficient and effective in distilling the essence of the cases, emphasizing the teaching points and helping the participants to become better healthcare providers by promoting positive teamwork and communication skills. Knowledge, attention to the cases and preparation prior to the competition will help you to be the best SimWars debriefer you can be.

BIBLIOGRAPHY

Fanning RM, Gaba DM. The role of debriefing in simulation-based learning. *Simul Healthc* 2007; 2:115–125.

Rudolph JW, Foldy EG, Robinson T. et al. Helping without harming: the instructor's feedback dilemma in debriefing – a case study. *Simul Healthc* 2013; 8:304–316.

Salas E, Klein C, King H et al. Debriefing medical teams: 12 evidence-based best practices and tips. *J Comm J Qual Patient Saf* 2008; 34:518–527.

CHAPTER 5

SimWars judging: maximizing the educational value of a popular modality

Scott D. Weingart and Jeremy Samuel Faust

Effective judging is a crucial component of the overall educational value of SimWars competitions for both the participants and the audience.

Unlike most forms of medical education evaluation, SimWars competitions are audited and often decided by a group of informed observers – the audience. The role of the judges is multifaceted. Judges must be at once didactic and frank with the teams while simultaneously influencing the audience's voting behavior in an effort to enhance the chance that the best team will emerge victorious. A SimWars judge must keep this in mind both in the formulation and in the subsequent delivery of constructive criticism. In sum, a successful SimWars judge provides insight, and often entertainment, in a remarkably confined time frame – frequently shorter than 90 seconds. This chapter offers several strategies that can be used for the successful execution of SimWars judging duties as a method for maximizing the educational impact of this increasingly popular and useful learning modality.

BREAKING DOWN JUDGING ROLES

SimWars judges are often chosen because of particular skills that they bring to the exercise. When possible, the judging panel should contain niche experts with complementary areas of knowledge with as little overlap as is feasible. This avoids repetition and increases opportunities for each judge to provide genuine insight to the competitors and observers. To further exploit the presence of judges with diverse areas of expertise, and to minimize repetition, judging panels should plan ahead and predetermine the niche that each judge will direct most of his or her attention during the evaluation and public debriefing. A medical education or simulation expert, for example, may be best suited to make comments related to the educational format itself, including teamwork, communication, delineation of roles and discussion of case summaries (more specific guidance is given in Chapter 4). This chapter will focus on judging clinical content.

JUDGING CLINICAL CONTENT

When possible, one judge should be chosen for each case to specifically focus on the clinical content and medical correctness of the team's treatment decisions and actions. This judge will often be a physician with advanced training or extensive experience in the case's focus and should be capable of dissecting the finer implications of medical decisions and actions taken as well as those that were missed.

When focusing on clinical content, we recommend addressing two main areas of a SimWars team's performance: assessment of the team's performance under pressure and of clinical correctness.

Performance under pressure. SimWars is the rare educational modality that tests quick, intuitive, heuristic and instinctual thinking, so-called "system 1/type 1" cognitive processes. In SimWars, stressors include the presence of the audience, constant pushing and distractions by actors, time constraints and the competitive nature of the experience – there are winners and losers. These elements were, in fact, designed to force "shoot-from-the-hip" thinking, in contrast to "system 2/ type 2" processes, in which decisions are made via slower, carefully considered and contemplative means. Therefore, unlike traditional didactic testing, Sim-Wars allows a unique and safe opportunity to evaluate a trainee's preparation for stressful complicated situations. Additionally, this set of crucial emergency medicine skills is often only otherwise on display for appraisal during the real-life management of unstable patients, which is not the optimal moment for thoughtful didactic observations by even the most experienced teacher. For more information on the types of cognitive behaviors that doctors display during decision making, we refer the reader directly to the work of Pat Croskerry, who has described multiple "cognitive dispositions to respond" as a scheme for demonstrating how doctors diagnose or fail to diagnose accurately, based on a variety of factors.

Clinical correctness of the team's performance. Evaluating teams for clinical competence may require up-close observation in order to overhear quieter team conversations that may be occurring in a potentially noisy SimWars environment. For this reason, and to evaluate the correctness of critical procedures (e.g. crichothyrotomy, thoracotomy, chest tube placement), a judge should feel free to roam from his or her seat in order to watch from up close, being careful not to disrupt the team or obstruct the audience's view for lengthy periods. (Teams should be warned that one judge may do this so they are not alarmed and jostled from their normal workflow.) Verifying that a procedure has been done correctly (e.g. assessing the size of an incision in a cricothyrotomy, observing how the trachea was dilated and confirming that the tube was correctly placed into the mannequin trachea) is an important and often overlooked component to judging a team's performance and important for assessing a team's competence to perform the procedure in a real-life case. The teams and the audience can benefit tremendously from these technical insights during the judges' debriefing comments. This is particularly important when a team's overall posture and flow appear to be smooth and well controlled in the eyes of the common observer. This can mislead the audience into the easy cognitive trap of mistaking comfort and confidence with correctness; a finely oiled SimWars machine can easily seduce an audience into falsely thinking that a case was handled optimally. The judge focusing on clinical content must consciously and openly address this during debriefing.

GIVING FEEDBACK

When done properly, debriefing can serve as both an educational and a recruiting opportunity, turning today's audience members into tomorrow's SimWars competitors. Providing effective feedback is a genuine and often acquired skill that is more difficult than typically acknowledged by teachers. In SimWars, this problem is magnified by the public component, as the learner is *exposed*. Indeed, by its very design, SimWars is not a *safe* learning environment. While this is one of SimWars' chief advantages (as it provides a pressure-filled testing ground for dangerous scenarios without actual lives being at stake), it can be a barrier for learning during debriefing if the judges shy away from being forthright. One way to decrease the emotional temperature while giving feedback is to be entertaining while providing honest insight. Here we will address some problems of providing public feedback as well as some observations on feedback delivery that can be applied in more traditional settings as well.

Giving feedback in public

A chief attribute shared by successful speeches and SimWars debriefings is brevity. Nothing breaks an audience's attention span more consistently than a meandering monologue. Being playful and entertaining while giving negative feedback not only delights the audience but can be a powerful device for defusing tension for the competitors. This may soften a judge's tougher criticisms. One simple yet effective disarming device is the use of familiar terms when addressing the competitors. "Adam, my friend, your incision was about an inch too small" is more effective than simply "That guy with the black hair really screwed up that cric."

A few other pointers on public feedback.

Avoid repetition. If a comment has already been made by another judge, do not repeat it. It is remarkable that many well-meaning judges will start a repetitive statement, "I don't want to be repetitive, however…," and then go on to be exactly that and "echo" the other judges' statements. The desire to double-up on a comment is particularly strong when you scribble down a particularly great teaching pearl during the case only to have a preceding judge hit that exact point. Avoiding this takes discipline but is beneficial for the flow of the competition and to keep the audience engaged.

Be brief. Generally, one judge per case should speak for a few minutes. The other judges should confine themselves to shorter comments, perhaps 60–90 seconds in length. Being pithy and efficient is a skill that can be developed with practice.

Practice. It is common to hear that someone does not like the sound of his or her own voice on recordings. Often, however, on close inspection, it is not the timbre or quality of the voice but rather it is having been forced to hear one's own suboptimal and jagged delivery of important content that people find so recoiling. This can be addressed by practicing in advance with an audio recorder. Many who do this will find that quality of delivery improves with practice. Over time, a rehearsed speaker may come to like the sound of his or her own voice on recordings. This is usually because the speaker has refined the delivery of his or her content, not because of improvements in their voice quality. Watching other judging competitions (such as televised talent and music shows) can be informative. These judges are professionals in the realm of being informative, entertaining and, above all else, brief.

Embrace disagreement. Not only does inter-judge disagreement demonstrate more than one successful approach to a difficult medical problem but audiences seem to love it when judges disagree. This adds an element to the fun of the competition and should be a welcome part of debriefing, provided that disagreements are respectful and the correct tone is maintained.

General strategies for giving effective feedback

As a panel, efforts must be taken to ensure that there is a balance between encouragement and criticism. In order to maximize the efficiency of the panel as a whole, one judge may be designated in advance to focus on negative parts of the team's performance while others may focus in on identifying strengths. This "good cop/bad cop" method has been exploited par excellence on television's "American Idol" for years and may serve as a good reference.

When delivering criticism, many teachers use the "feedback sandwich" method. In this method, compliments at the beginning and end of the debriefing (the "bread") surround the main criticisms (the "meat"). This can be effective. However, students predisposed to be overconfident may only focus on the bread; less confident students may only focus on the meat. The main problem with the "feedback sandwich," however, is that it often fails to provide the recipients with an accurate sense of their overall performance and leaves them without a plan of remediating action. Another problem is that certain judges may attempt to deliver the "feedback sandwich" but in the end may be unable to resist opening with and at the end recapitulating the negative comments – the "inside-out feedback sandwich." This can be all too tempting for the judge who holds particularly high standards and is passionate about demanding high-quality performances from learners.

For these reasons, we recommend consideration of the "GRIP" scheme during debriefing: grade, reassurance, insight, prognostication. In this scheme, an overall "grade" is immediately stated (poor, satisfactory, very good, excellent). This is followed by "reassurance," a positive observation of something that went well. This sets up a safer environment for the delivery of "insight," usually the most important part of the critique in which negative criticism is proffered. Finally, during "prognostication," substantive suggestions are offered as well as a prediction of how the team would fare if they were able to successfully incorporate this advice. For example:

> I thought the overall performance was very good. You correctly diagnosed an unstable and then crashing patient with upper GI bleeding. You appropriately progressed towards a cricothyrotomy when other options failed. However, your incision was not in the correct place and was not the correct length, resulting in incorrect tube placement. The correct incision should have been larger and more inferior on the mannequin anatomy. Despite your correct decision making, this error alone would have cost the patient's life. If your team improves on the finer points of your procedural skills, I believe your overall performance has the potential to progress from very good to excellent.

SUMMARY

The SimWars modality is a valuable training ground for the assessment of heuristic thinking, teamwork, quick decision making and medical knowledge. Judges with complementary niches of clinical expertise should be represented on the panel in order to provide the most insight to the competitors and the audience; this should include at least one evaluator focusing on clinical content and correctness of each case. Effective debriefing is a form of public speaking and should be treated as such by practicing in advance in order to achieve delivery of balanced but insightful feedback in a useful manner.

BIBLIOGRAPHY

Croskerry P. The importance of cognitive errors in diagnosis and strategies to minimize them. *Acad Med* 2003; 78:775–780.

Croskerry P. Diagnostic failure: a cognitive and affective approach. In Henriksen K, Battles JB, Marks ES, et al., eds. *Advances in Patient Safety: From Research to Implementation: Vol 2 Concepts and Methodology*. Rockville, MD: Agency for Healthcare Research and Quality, Rockville, MD: Agency for Healthcare Research and Quality, 2005, 2005.

Stanovich KE. *Who is Rational? Studies of Individual Differences in Reasoning*. Mahwah, NJ: Erlbaum, 1999.

CHAPTER 6

Troubleshooting technology

Lisa Jacobson

This chapter discusses how to address issues that occur with technology. Most people who have worked with a simulator (or any technology) understand at times the machine may not do what you want. A general rule in SimWars is "if it's broken for team A, it's broken for team B." Realistically, practitioners will experience broken light sources while intubating, missing vital sign tracings on the monitor or difficult exams and adapt accordingly. At various points in SimWars competitions, this has happened by accident, but as long as the competition is kept consistent it has not been a problem. Again, here is where having a well-versed facilitator involved in the scenario can help in maintaining the participant's suspension of disbelief. A quick reply of "I see the monitor is not working doctor, I will see if I can get another" avoids distracting further from the competition even though adding another degree of difficulty.

When SimWars has been held in large hotels or conference centers, wireless internet interference has also complicated the production. Often the audiovisual staff at the location can provide information as to whether they have wireless signal blocking at their institution or multiple sources of wireless signal, either of which can complicate using a wireless simulator and may require machines to be run wired. As venues for SimWars have expanded, the need for lavalier microphones for participants and, importantly, someone to manage their output, has grown. Microphone interference is not something that augments the desired realism in simulation. Most importantly, acknowledging the limitations in any technology before beginning will aid in preparing for those challenges in advance. This forethought will improve production of the scenarios and avoid the potential pitfall of complete reliance on technology for success. Preserving suspension of disbelief optimizes team and individual performance and is, therefore, critical for the success of any SimWars competition.

PART II

SIMWARS CASES

SECTION 1

AIRWAY MANAGEMENT

Terminal extubation

Lisa Jacobson

1. SCENARIO OVERVIEW

EMS brings in a 75-year-old female resuscitated in the field, now intubated with return of spontaneous circulation (ROSC). Patient has metastatic breast cancer, is on palliative chemotherapy and collapsed at home. A neighbor called 911 and EMS arrived and initiated care, regaining VS after intubation and a round of epinephrine. Initial rhythm was PEA. Phone rings after 1 minute, while team is initiating care in the ED and family reports that they have found the DNR/DNI paperwork that they did not present to the EMS team and demand that the doctor remove the tube immediately as the patient never wanted this. Team will have to terminally extubate the patient.

2. TEACHING OBJECTIVES/DISCUSSION POINTS

Actions related to advanced directives

- Confirm paperwork, correct identities
- Confirm intent of the paperwork
- Discuss with family what this means today explicitly
- Address dissenting family member's concerns

Actions related to palliation

- Opioid drip
- Sedative drip if deemed necessary

Actions related to extubation

- Methods include withdrawal of ventilation not intubation, T-tube, or just extubating and then humidified O_2
- Secretion control: glycopyrrolate or atropine

3. SUPPLIES

Mannequin, ETT with ventilator tubing, IV supplies.

4. MOULAGE

Make-up for elderly, pale, ill-appearing patient, women's gray wig, fluids for secretions.

5. IMAGES AND LABS

■ XR26: CXR with right mainstem intubation
■ Advanced directive/AND/DNR paperwork

6. ACTORS (CONFEDERATES) AND THEIR ROLES

■ EMS: brings in the patient already intubated and report resuscitation and ROSC.
■ Nurse: helpful, expresses concern about pain, suffering, legality of documents.
■ Family members: provide AND/DNR paperwork, mainly supportive pushing for terminal extubation with the exception of a cousin who does not want to wean.

7. CRITICAL ACTIONS

■ Determine advanced directive
■ Initiate family discussion
■ Terminal extubation
■ Manage pain
■ Manage secretions

8. TIMELINE

Time 0

VS: BP 90/65, HR 110, RR, EMS bagging, O_2 Sat 95% (tubed) (although not initially on monitor: case starts as patient is wheeled in door)

■ IV access in right antecubital fossa, 20G
■ EKG monitor: sinus tachycardia 110
■ Physical exam
  ▶ General: unresponsive, cachectic, in her pajamas
  ▶ HEENT: pupils fixed and dilated, tube in place at 26 cm at lip
  ▶ Chest: decreased bowel sounds on left
  ▶ Heart: regular, tachy
  ▶ Abdomen: soft
  ▶ Skin: no other injuries, warm, dry
  ▶ Extremities: no injuries noted, leg edema
  ▶ Neuro: fixed, dolls eyes, no gag
■ Nurse cue: "let's get this patient on the vent so we can stop bagging"
■ EMS cue: "we'd like to get out of here, can we have our lifepack back"

Critical actions
● Confirm ETT placement
● Set ventilator

Transition point 1: 1 minute

■ BP 90/65, HR 110, RR: set by team Sat 91%; vent alarming unless tube already adjusted
■ Phone call from family – there is a DNR/DNI – we're on our way
■ Vent continues to alarm unless ETT is readjusted from mainstem position
■ Cue from Nurse: "what's that beeping? Did you confirm placement? I don't hear breath sounds on the left"

Critical actions
● Adjust ETT
● Address alarming vent

Transition point 2: 2 minutes

■ BP 90/65, HR 110, RR set by team O_2 Sat 95% if ETT adjusted
■ Family arrives
  ▶ "She doesn't want the tube in"
  ▶ "We told the ambulance she didn't want any aggressive measures"
  ▶ one verbal cousin disagrees, wants everything done
■ XR26 is available (XR3 if readjusted)

Critical actions
● Confirm DNR
● Address family concerns/dissent

Transition point 3: 4 minutes

VS unchanged

■ Family continues to vocalize how this isn't what she'd want, take out the tube:
  ▶ family member calls in – daughter is a endocrinologist attending at a hospital in Virginia – has questions about patient's exam, why she coded
  ▶ family demanding extubation, does not accept "we don't do that here" as an excuse
  ▶ if team flat refuses to extubate, the PMD calls in having just received a call from the family to advocate for extubation as well
■ Nurse and family begin to worry about pain and suffering if team has not started opioid drip:
  ▶ "All she wanted was to be comfortable"
  ▶ "She takes so much pain medicine at home"

Critical actions
● Confirm surrogates
● Discuss concerns with family/PMD
● Address pain

Transition point 4: final actions

VS unchanged

- ■ End case with either extubation or family satisfaction with no extubation
    - ▶ family only satisfied if there is a plan for extubation
    - ▶ may be waiting for clergy
    - ▶ pain and suffering addressed
- ■ Disposition: non-ICU setting if extubated
    - ▶ involve clergy, palliative care, hospice care if possible

Critical actions
- Facilitate family discussion
- Manage secretions
- Discuss options for wean
- Consult clergy etc.

9. STIMULI

- ■ XR26: CXR with right mainstem intubation
- ■ DNR/AND appropriate to your facility

10. BIBLIOGRAPHY

Kompanje EJ et al. Anticipation of distress after discontinuation of mechanical ventilation in the ICU at the end of life. *Intensive Care Med* 2008; 34:1593–1599.

Limehouse WE et al. A model for emergency department end-of-life communications after acute devastating events. Part I: decision-making capacity, surrogates, and advanced directives. *Acad Emerg Med* 2012;19(9):E1068–E1072.

Mazer MA et al. The infusion of opioids during terminal withdrawal of mechanical ventilation in the medical intensive care unit. *J Pain Symptom Manage* 2011; 42:44–51.

Industrial fire victim: burns and cyanide toxicity

Scott Goldberg and Steven A. Godwin

1. SCENARIO OVERVIEW

A 35-year-old man presents to the ED, a victim of an industrial fire. Apparently, a colleague arrived to work to find the building on fire. He ran in to find his friend unconscious with debris on top of him. He dragged the patient to his personal vehicle and brought him to the ED. The patient has sustained burns to his upper chest, back and circumferentially around left arm. On ED arrival he is moaning in pain.

2. TEACHING OBJECTIVES/DISCUSSION POINTS

Clinical and medical management

- Appropriate management of burns involving the airway
- Appropriate analgesia and fluid resuscitation of a severely burned patient
- Consider the indications for cyanide antidote in burns
- Consider carbon monoxide toxicity in burns and smoke inhalation

Communication and teamwork

- Work as a team to appropriately manage a patient with complicated burns
- Appropriate and timely discussion with a burn referral center for patient transfer

3. SUPPLIES

Burned overalls or shirt, singed wig, model hydroxycobalamin antidote kit.

4. MOULAGE

Soot around mouth and nares, singed hair, burnt overalls or shirt, circumferential burns to chest wall and left arm.

5. IMAGES AND LABS

- XR1: normal male CXR
- XR3: normal male intubated CXR

■ EKG1: sinus tachycardia
■ US1: normal FAST
■ Labs: ABG, carboxyhemoglobin, lactate

6. ACTORS (CONFEDERATES) AND THEIR ROLES

■ Nurse: generally helpful; may prompt team to transfer patient to a center with burn services.
■ Friend: provides limited information but generally helpful and non-obstructive.
■ Toxicology consult: will suggest empiric hydroxycobalamin based on lactate level.
■ Burn center: will accept transfer of patient, will arrange hyperbarics if requested.

7. CRITICAL ACTIONS

■ Consider potential additional traumatic injuries
■ Identify a potentially difficult airway and manage appropriately
■ Adequate analgesia and fluid resuscitation
■ Empiric treatment of cyanide toxicity
■ Identify and manage of potential carbon monoxide toxicity

8. TIMELINE

Time 0

VS: BP 160/95, HR 130, RR 20, O_2 Sat 92% RA, 36.9°C, EKG – sinus tachycardia

■ Prehospital interventions: none
■ Physical exam
  ▶ General: semi-alert, in severe pain, with soot around mouth and nares; moaning
  ▶ PMH: unknown
  ▶ Past sexual history: unknown
  ▶ Social history: unknown
  ▶ Medication: unknown
  ▶ Allergies: NKDA
  ▶ HEENT: Pupils 2 mm and reactive; singed hair around nares and mouth; no soot in mouth; no appreciable edema of lips or tongue
  ▶ Neck: supple; some faint stridor
  ▶ Chest: clear to auscultation; second-degree burns of chest wall
  ▶ Heart: regular rhythm, tachycardia
  ▶ Back: second-degree burns
  ▶ Abdomen: normal
  ▶ Extremities: second-degree burns circumferentially around left arm; pulses symmetric
  ▶ Skin: diaphoretic
  ▶ Neuro: only moaning to pain; responds to painful stimuli; opens eyes spontaneously

▶ Total body surface area burned: 25%
▶ Glucose: 110
■ Friend: very upset, "If only I had gotten there sooner!" "Is he going to be OK?"
■ Nurse: generally helpful, no trouble gaining IV access

Critical actions
- Identify a critical trauma patient and begin assessment
- Begin consideration of airway management
- Identify potential for additional traumatic injuries
- Obtain blood work including carboxyhemoglobin and lactate levels

Transition point 1: 2 minutes

VS: BP 115/70, HR 140, RR 20, O_2 Sat 90% RA, 94% NRB

■ IV fluids and analgesia will decrease the heart rate somewhat
■ If attempts are made to intubate: move to next transition
■ Team should complete secondary assessment
■ IV fluids should be administered
■ Transfer should be considered for burn center/hyperbarics
■ FAST: negative
■ Labs: ABG, carboxyhemoglobin
■ Nurse: if team tried to consult burn or trauma service, these teams are not available at this hospital. If they want to transfer then the nurse will put in a page to the local receiving center

Critical actions
- Secondary survey
- Appropriate fluid resuscitation for an approximately 25% total body surface burn
- Continued analgesia
- Consideration of carbon monoxide poisoning
- Consideration of transfer

Transition point 2: 4 minutes

VS: BP 80/50, HR 135, RR 35, O_2 Sat 70% RA, 85% NRB

■ Voice becomes muffled, drooling, stridor
■ If team elects to intubate via direct laryngoscopy:
    ▶ patient is unable to be intubated
    ▶ patient will require cricothyroidotomy
■ If team elects to intubate using fiberoptic or awake technique:
    ▶ intubation is successful
■ Labs: lactate
■ Imaging: CXR
■ Friend: if team has not secured airway, friend begins to ask "why does he sound different"

> **Critical actions**
> - Airway management, preferably with advanced airway approach
> - Begin post-intubation management
> - Consideration of cyanide toxicity

Transition point 3: final actions

VS: BP 60/30, HR 150, on ventilation, O_2 Sat 88% (on ventilation)

■ Administration of cyanide antidote will improve BP to 90/50
■ If team administers vasopressors, BP will improve appropriate to medication and dosing chosen
■ Continued post-intubation management
■ If team has not already administered cyanide antidote it should be hung
■ Toxicology: will recommend appropriate dosing of hydroxycobalamin if consulted
■ Burn center: will accept transfer of patient, will be able to arrange for hyperbarics if requested. Recommend cyanide antidote if it has not been given

> **Critical actions**
> - Continued post-intubation care
> - Administration of cyanide antidote
> - Appropriate disposition to burn center

9. STIMULI

■ XR1: normal male CXR
■ XR3: normal intubated male CXR
■ US1: normal FAST
■ Labs:
  ▶ pH 7.05
  ▶ PCO_2 46 mmHg
  ▶ PO_2 286 mmHg
  ▶ Bicarbonate 8
  ▶ Sat 85%
  ▶ Carboxyhemoglobin 19%
  ▶ Lactate 10.4 mmol/L

10. BIBLIOGRAPHY

Edlich RF, Martin ML, Long WB 3rd. Thermal burns. In Marx JA, Hockberger RS, Walls RM, eds. Rosen's Emergency Medicine: Concepts and Clinical Practice, 6th edn. Philadelphia, PA: Mosby Elsevier, 2006, Ch. 60.

Gómez R, Cancio LC. Management of burn wounds in the emergency department. *Emerg Med Clin North Am* 2007; 25:135–146.

Hettiaratchy S, Papini R. Initial management of a major burn: I – overview. *BMJ* 2004; 328:1555–1557.

O'Brien DJ, Walsh DW, Terriff CM, Hall AH. Empiric management of cyanide toxicity associated with smoke inhalation. *Prehosp Disaster Med* 2011; 26:374–382.

Schwartz L, Balakrishnan C. Thermal burns. In Tintinalli JE, Kelen GD, Stapczynski JS, eds. *Emergency Medicine: A Comprehensive Study Guide*, 6th edn. New York: McGraw-Hill, 2004, Ch. 199.

Pool diving accident

Neal Aaron and Steven A. Godwin

1. SCENARIO OVERVIEW

A 24-year-old man presents after a pool diving accident. Friends, who had all been drinking with the patient, report that he jumped into a shallow swimming pool and was thought to be playing at the bottom of the pool for approximately 3–4 minutes before he was pulled from the pool in apparent cardiac arrest. A paramedic at the scene initiated bystander CPR and the patient had ROSC at rescue's arrival 5 minutes later. Rescue gave the patient a GCS of 3. The patient's airway was managed with a King LT at the scene.

2. TEACHING OBJECTIVES/DISCUSSION POINTS

Clinical and medical management

- Recognition of neurogenic shock
- Management of neurogenic shock
- Evaluation of potential head trauma
- Management of post-traumatic patients with cardiac arrest and hypothermia: what to do when the etiology is not clear
- Airway management with c-spine injury and supraglottic device
    ▶ recognition of potential for swelling and airway compromise

3. SUPPLIES

- Cervical collar
- Cooling blanket
- IV fluids
- King LT (or other supraglottic airway)
- PEEP valve, airway supplies

4. MOULAGE

Mannequin in swimming attire with c-collar in place, King LT tube (laryngeal tube), small abrasion of top of forehead.

5. IMAGES AND LABS

■ XR5: male CXR intubated with aspiration
■ CT1: normal head CT
■ CT2: c-spine with high fracture
■ XR6: lateral c-spine with high cervical fracture and with significant intrusion on the cord
■ EKG2: normal sinus rhythm

6. ACTORS (CONFEDERATES) AND THEIR ROLES

■ Patient: mannequin, non-responsive.
■ Nurse: assist with tasks as assigned by team leader.
■ MICU consult: available as a voice.

7. CRITICAL ACTIONS

■ Post-arrest assessment
  ▶ tube confirmation, securing
  ▶ rhythm analysis
■ Trauma exam and assessment
■ Exchange King LT for definitive airway
■ Recognize and treat neurogenic shock
■ Discuss and/or implement hypothermia protocol
■ Ventilate drowning victim

8. TIMELINE

Time 0

VS: BP 90/50, HR 76, RR 16, O_2 Sat 99% BVM, 96°F, EKG – sinus rhythm at 76

■ Patient is unresponsive
■ 18 gauge IV catheter in right forearm placed by EMS
■ Physical exam
  ▶ General: supraglottic device in place, unresponsive
  ▶ HEENT: 4 mm and minimally reactive
  ▶ Neck: step-off at C3
  ▶ Chest: coarse bowel sounds bilaterally, worse on right
  ▶ Heart: regular rate and rhythm without m/r/g
  ▶ Abdomen: mildly distended but soft, bowel sounds hypoactive
  ▶ Rectal: no tone, no gross blood
  ▶ Skin: moist, abrasion on top of forehead
  ▶ Extremities: no signs of trauma
  ▶ Neuro: unresponsive; GCS 5 (eyes 1, voice 1, motor 3, decorticate posturing)
  ▶ FAST: normal (US1) if done

Transition point 1: 1 minute

VS: BP 90/50, HR 76, RR 16, O_2 Sat 99% BVM

■ Changes in physical exam: none
■ Labs: none available
■ Imaging: none available

Critical actions
- Replace King LT with definitive airway. No glidescope or fiberoptics available
- RSI with cervical spine precautions
- Use neuroprotective RSI: consider reduced induction doses even with etomidate otherwise BP will worsen further

---

Transition point 2: 3 minutes

VS: BP 65/40, HR 76, RR 16, O_2 Sat 100% BVM

■ Begins to demonstrate *more* hypotension regardless of induction agent
■ If IV fluids given, BP does not change. Once 2 L IV fluids given, initiate pressors for neurogenic shock. If no IV fluids, systolic BP drops to 50s over the next 2 minutes
■ If airway controlled and fluids/pressors given for neurogenic shock, will need CT head and CT c-spine
■ Labs: none available
■ Imaging: none available
■ Nurse (confederate 1): helpful, completes assigned tasks

Critical actions
- Volume resuscitation
- Initiation of pressors after 2–3 L

Transition point 3: 6 minutes

VS: unchanged

■ If airway controlled and fluids/pressors given for neurogenic shock, will need CT head and CT c-spine
■ Labs
  ▶ Chem-7: normal
  ▶ CBC: normal
  ▶ PT/PTT/INR: normal
  ▶ Urine DOA: +marijuana, otherwise negative
  ▶ Blood alcohol: 267
■ Imaging available
  ▶ CT1: normal CT head
  ▶ CT2, c-spine CT with high fracture
  ▶ XR6: lateral c-spine with high cervical fracture (C3) with significant intrusion on the cord
■ Nurse (confederate 1): points out shock if team has yet to manage it; nurse recognizes frothy sputum from ETT

Critical actions
- CT head and c-spine
- Post-intubation hypoxia management with placement of PEEP valve to improve O_2 saturation

Transition point 4: final actions

VS: BP 110/72, HR 88, RR 16 at 84–88%

- Difficulty maintaining O_2 saturation due to frothy edema
- Address hypothermia protocol (MICU consultant will ask if not already done)
- Disposition: admit to MICU
- Neurosurgeon (confederate 2): is abrupt but will accept consult, recommends admission to ICU
- ICU consultant (confederate 3): accepts patient

Critical actions
- Initiate hypothermia protocol; at minimum cold fluid bolus and ask to begin protocol
- Consult neurosurgery or spine
- MICU admission

9. STIMULI

- XR5: male CXR intubated with aspiration
- CT1: normal head CT
- CT2: c-spine CT with high fracture
- XR6: lateral c-spine with high cervical fracture and with significant intrusion on the cord
- EKG2: normal sinus rhythm

10. BIBLIOGRAPHY

Baron BJ, McSherry KJ, Larson, JL, Jr., Scalea TM. Spine and spinal cord trauma. In Tintinalli JE, Stapczynski JS, Cline DM et al. eds. Tintinalli's Emergency Medicine: A Comprehensive Study Guide, 7th edn. New York: McGraw-Hill, 2011, Ch. 255.

Consortium for Spinal Cord Medicine. Early acute management in adults with spinal cord injury: a clinical practice guideline for health-care professionals. *J Spinal Cord Med* 2008;31:403–479.

Gupta M, Benson D, Keenan T. Initial evaluation and emergency treatment of the spine-injured patient. In Browner BD ed. *Skeletal Trauma*, 4th edn. Philapelphia, PA: Saunders-Elsevier, 2009, Ch. 25.

CASE 4

Difficult airway: house fire

Kristin McKee and Steven A. Godwin

1. SCENARIO OVERVIEW

A 35-year-old man presents after crawling under his house and setting himself on fire after an argument with his girlfriend. A passerby saw him and rushed to pull him out. He presents with major burn injury below his neck and loud, noisy breathing. Patient will be hypoxic and have a difficult airway. If RSI is preformed, the patient will need to have a cricothyrotomy performed. After intubation, the patient will remain hypoxic secondary to cyanide toxicity and need for an escharotomy. Once these actions are complete the patient will be transferred to a burn center.

2. TEACHING OBJECTIVES/DISCUSSION POINTS

Clinical and medical management

■ Difficult airway recognition and management
■ Recognition and management of cyanide poisoning
■ Performance of an escharotomy

3. SUPPLIES

Burn mock-up allowing for escharotomy. IV fluids, cricothyrotomy set-up, basic IV and airway supplies.

4. MOULAGE

Full-thickness burns circumferential to bilateral thighs, stomach and chest; deep and superficial partial thickness to bilateral arms and neck.

5. IMAGES AND LABS

■ XR1: normal male CXR
■ XR3: normal intubated male CXR
■ EKG1: sinus tachycardia

6. ACTORS (CONFEDERATES) AND THEIR ROLES

▓ EMS: gives summary of what happened; this starts at time 0.
▓ Nurse: delivers medications and draws labs.
▓ Patient: struggles to breathe and moans, has stridor.
▓ Consult: burn doctor takes report.

7. CRITICAL ACTIONS

▓ Identify the difficult airway
▓ Manage the difficult airway
▓ Identify cyanide poisoning
▓ Manage cyanide poisoning
▓ Manage burns
▓ Perform chest and leg escharotomies
▓ Transfer to burn center

8. TIMELINE

Time 0

VS: BP 135/90, pulse 120, HR 26, 98°F, O_2 Sat 75% RA, EKG: sinus rhythm at 120

▓ Summary of initial presentation: 35-year-old man presents after crawling under his house and setting himself on fire; was pulled out by passerby. Presents with major burn injury below his neck and loud, noisy breathing. He is moaning and sounds stridorous.
▓ Initial interventions: IV placed by rescue, 18G forearm
▓ Physical exam
  ▶ General: tearful and alert but struggling to breath and moaning in pain
  ▶ HEENT: pupils 4 mm and reactive
  ▶ Neck: supple
  ▶ Chest: limited air movement, stridorous sounds
  ▶ Heart: tachycardic without murmur
  ▶ Abdomen: soft, non-tender, normal bowel sounds
  ▶ Skin: full-thickness burns circumferential to bilateral thighs, stomach and chest, deep and superficial partial thickness to bilateral arms and neck
  ▶ Extremities: poor perfusion of bilateral lower extremities
  ▶ Neuro: alert, able to grip bilaterally, moves all extremities with pain
▓ Nurse (confederate): must facilitate exam findings on mannequin

Critical action
- Identify difficult airway
- ATLS

Transition point 1: 2 minutes

▓ Vitals unchanged, worsening stridor
▓ Airway assessment

- Additional access not available, labs drawn from EMS line
- Intubation:
  - if "awake" or facilitated look: will be able to intubate
  - if RSI, will have failed airway and will need to perform a cricothyrotomy
- Post-confirmed intubation: CO_2 exchange, breath sounds difficult to assess with burns, O_2 Sat remains in low 80s

Critical action
- Manage difficult airway and confirm tube placement

Transition point 2: 4 minutes

VS: BP 135/90, P120, HR 26, 98°F, O_2 Sat 80% on 100% FiO_2

- Recognize and treat CN toxicity
  - if antidote given saturation slowly improves to 100% on FiO_2 100%
- initiate fluid resuscitation using Parkland formula or maintaining urine output
- CXR available

Critical action
- Identifiy and manage cyanide toxicity
- Fluid resuscitation

Transition point 3: final actions

VS: BP 135/90, pulse 120, HR 26, 98°F, O_2 Sat 84–88% on 100% FiO_2

- Saturation declines again if had improved after appropriate antidote
- Becomes more difficult to ventilate
- Escharotomy necessary for ventilation, possibly for perfusion of lower extremities
- Labs:
  - Chem 7: normal
  - CBC: normal
  - carboxyhemoglobin
- Burn doctor (confederate): accepts transfer if team can coherently present case; otherwise will probe for toxicology details and airway ventilation challenges

Critical action
- Perform chest and leg escharotomies
- Transfer to burn center

9. STIMULI

- XR1: normal male CXR
- XR3: normal male intubated CXR
- EKG1: sinus tachycardia

10. BIBLIOGRAPHY

Gomez R, Cancio L. Management of burn wounds in the emergency department. *Emerg Med Clinics North Am* 2007;25:135–146.

Orgill DP. Escharotomy and decompressive therapies in burns. *J Burn Care Res* 2009; 30: 759–768.

"Is there a doctor on the plane?": airplane anaphylaxis

Brandon J. Godbout and Jessica Hernandez

1. SCENARIO OVERVIEW

A team of learners are seated sporadically in rows, resembling those of an airplane, amongst random audience members, and are called to action to the panicked overhead announcement: "Is there a doctor on the plane?" Team members find a 17-year-old woman with a history of panic attacks and peanut anaphylaxis in the past, allergy information *not* volunteered, complaining of shortness of breath and lightheadedness while on a flight, midway from New York City to San Diego. They need to tease out the information that she was eating plane cookies (on back of package states: *may contain peanuts*) while inflight and shortly after feels chest and throat tightness, as well as shortness of breath. Over time she becomes more flushed, itchy, wheezy and agitated. Additionally, a non-medical passenger becomes obstructive to the team during inflight resuscitation. The patient will remain critical, but stable, if appropriate treatment is administered *and* pilot is directed to immediately land the flight. The patient will decompensate to complete upper airway obstruction and respiratory arrest if either of these do not occur.

2. TEACHING OBJECTIVES/DISCUSSION POINTS

Clinical and medical management

- Identify anaphylaxis
- Appropriately manage anaphylaxis with limited resources
- Demonstrate knowledge of basic and advanced airplane medical kits
- Understand indications for immediate flight landing

Communication and teamwork

- Orchestrate an effective team model in a chaotic and unfamiliar environment
- Demonstrate timely and effective removal of an obstructive bystander
- Appropriate and frequent communication of patient status with flight personnel and pilot

3. SUPPLIES

▉ *Basic inflight medical kit*
  ▶ sphygmomanometer
  ▶ stethoscope
  ▶ gloves
  ▶ thermometer
  ▶ bandages
▉ *Advanced inflight medical kit (quantity of item)*
  ▶ aspirin 325 mg tablets (4)
  ▶ diphenhydramine 25 mg tablets (4) and 50 mg IV ampules (2)
  ▶ D50/50 mL IV ampule (1)
  ▶ epinephrine 1:1000 (2 single dose ampules)
  ▶ epinephrine 1:10 000 (2 ampules of 2 mL)
  ▶ albuterol MDI (1)
  ▶ lidocaine 20 mg/mL (2 ampules of 5 mL)
  ▶ nitroglycerin 0.4 mg sl tablets (10)
  ▶ Normal saline (a 500 mL bag)
  ▶ AED
  ▶ O_2 source
  ▶ oropharyngeal airways (3 sizes)
  ▶ syringes
  ▶ needles
  ▶ IV tubing
  ▶ AMBU bag (3 sizes of mask)
▉ *Other supplies*
  ▶ Prescription bottle with 12 prednisone tablets (20 mg each; from an asthmatic passenger), background screen projector, seats, stewardess outfit, mannequin outfitted in normal clothes, female wig, ballpoint pen

4. MOULAGE

Make-up (urticaria), liquid latex (lip swelling).

5. IMAGES AND LABS

Image of airplane cabin (for overhead projector), audio file of airplane cabin noise (to be played in background throughout case): not provided

6. ACTORS (CONFEDERATES) AND THEIR ROLES

▉ Flight attendant: responsible for facilitating retrieval of medical kits (only brings advanced inflight medical kit if requested). If team does not specify, stewardess brings the basic kit.
▉ Pilot (overhead voice only): to communicate status of patient and need for landing. Will push team to continue flying to destination (approximately 3 hours more) unless absolutely necessary.

■ Obstructive passenger: attempts to supersede team leader and interrupt team communication and resuscitation by repetitively stating, "she (patient) must have a collapsed lung, we need to put a needle in her chest" (despite having equal and normal breath sounds bilaterally). Team attempts to understand thought process but passenger becomes uncompromisingly agitated and attempts to manage situation him/herself. Team concludes that this passenger has no medical credentials (despite knowing some medicine) and is acting somewhat neurotically and will need to organize a strategic plan to remove obstructive passenger from resuscitation area.

■ Other passengers (optional): used to fill seats, depending on how many chairs. One passenger is an asthmatic and holds in possession a bottle of prednisone "in case of an asthma exacerbation." Team would need to seek out and ask passengers if they have any medicines that may be helpful (not included in the medical kits) in order to obtain and use the steroid.

7. CRITICAL ACTIONS

■ Obtain appropriate history and physical exam information related to complaint of shortness of breath and identify cause being secondary to anaphylaxis

■ Demonstrate accurate medical knowledge, including prompt treatment of anaphylaxis with O_2, epinephrine, diphenhydramine, albuterol, IV fluids and steroids (optional, if obtained), and proper medication dosage, particularly epinephrine concentration, dose and route

■ Utilize resources effectively in an unfamiliar environment, including knowledge of different medical kits

■ Communicate effectively within the team and with other passengers, including non-confrontational attempts to remove obstructive bystander

■ Work together to manage difficult case

■ Instruct pilot adamantly to land airplane at nearest airport for further management of stable but critical patient, knowing condition is potentially life threatening, progressive, time dependent and/or beyond scope of in-flight treatment only

8. TIMELINE

Time 0

VS: BP 100/55, HR 124, RR 28, O_2 Sat not available, 38.7°C

■ Summary of initial presentation: 17-year-old female seat-belted in airplane chair with normal clothes, cookie wrapper on lap and in moderate respiratory distress; slight flushing of neck

■ Initial interventions: none

■ Stewardess: assists in evaluation of patient

■ Physical exam
  ▶ General: anxious appearing, slightly tachypneic, speaking full sentences
  ▶ HEENT: minimal-mild swelling of lips and uvula, no stridor
  ▶ Neck: slightly flushed at collar line
  ▶ Chest: mild bilateral wheezing, tachycardic

▶ Abdomen: normal
▶ Skin: chest/neck skin flushed with occasional urticaria under clothes
▶ Neuro: normal

> **Critical actions**
> - Assess ABCs
> - Obtain history
> - Perform physical examination
> - Apply O_2

Transition point 1: 2 minutes

VS: BP 100/55, HR 124, RR 28, O_2 Sat not available, 38.7°C

■ Physical exam: no changes from initial exam (patient remains stable)
■ Stewardess: offers basic medical kit (if not requested)

> **Critical actions**
> - Obtain basic medical kit
> - Identify anaphylaxis
> - Communicate evaluation with flight team

Transition point 2: 5 minutes (deterioration point)

VS: BP 85/45, HR 134, RR 32 Sat (N/A), 38.7°C

■ Changes in physical exam/patient condition:
▶ General: moderate tachypneic, speaking 2–3 words at a time, panicked, upset by obstructive passenger
▶ HEENT: mild-moderate swelling of lips and uvula, patent airway
▶ Neck: flushed
▶ Chest: extensive bilateral wheezing, tachycardic
▶ Abdomen: normal
▶ Skin: completely flushed
▶ Neuro: tremulous
■ Stewardess: obtains advanced medical kit (if requested). If advanced kit not requested by 5-minute mark, stewardess prompts team, "Can I get any other equipment?"
■ Obstructive passenger: begins questioning team's knowledge and management decisions. States repetitively "I think she has a collapsed lung"

> **Critical actions**
> - Obtain advanced medical kit
> - Give epinephrine
> - Give other medication (i.e. diphenhydramine, albuterol)
> - Establish IV access and give IV fluids
> - Appropriately attempt talking down obstructive bystander

Transition point 3: 7 minutes

VS: BP 90/50, HR 125, RR 24, O_2 Sat not available, 38.7°C

■ Changes in physical exam/patient condition: if appropriate medications given, wheezing will improve and patient will be less agitated (critical but more stable)
■ Stewardess: if discussion regarding landing plane does not occur by 7-minute mark, stewardess prompts team, "Now that she is okay, we can continue to San Diego, correct? We see panic attacks on the plane all the time."
■ Obstructive passenger: becomes increasingly obstructive and louder. At times trying to force way towards patient and interfering with team dynamics
■ Other passenger (if not prompted): "I have prednisone for asthma, do you need it?"
■ Patient will deteriorate to complete airway obstruction if advanced medical kit not obtained and epinephrine not given by 6-minute mark. Seconds after complete airway obstruction cardiovascular collapse will occur. Heroic measures (i.e. ball-point pen cricothyroidotomy) will not change status, patient will die and case will end

Critical actions
- Reassess vital signs
- Inquire if another passenger is carrying medicine (steroid)
- Initiate discussion regarding landing plane with pilot
- Remove obstructive passenger from scene

Transition point 4: final actions

VS: BP 90/50, HR 125, RR 24, O_2 Sat not available, 38.7°C

■ Changes in physical exam/patient condition:
  ▶ General: less anxious appearing, slightly tachypneic, speaking full sentences
  ▶ HEENT: minimal–mild swelling of lips and uvula, no stridor
  ▶ Neck: no more flushing
  ▶ Chest: mild bilateral wheezing, tachycardic
  ▶ Abdomen: normal
  ▶ Skin: rare hive persists
  ▶ Neuro: normal
■ Stewardess: "Are you sure we need to land the plane?"
■ Obstructive passenger: no longer part of the case

Critical actions
- Reassure patient
- Mandate plane landing
- Communicate status with ground medical-control

9. STIMULI

None provided.

10. BIBLIOGRAPHY

Gendreau M and C DeJohn. Responding to medical events during commercial airline flights. *N Engl J Med* 2002; 346:1067–1073.

Kanwar M, C Irvin, J Frank et al. Confusion about epinephrine dosing leading to iatrogenic overdose: a life-threatening problem with a potential solution. *Ann Emerg Med* 2010; 55: 341–344.

SECTION 2

ALTERED MENTAL STATUS

Hyperthermia on a cruise ship

Jessica Hernandez and Jacqueline A. Nemer

1. SCENARIO OVERVIEW

This is a hybrid simulation case that begins with an actor and switches to a manne-quin when the patient becomes unresponsive. Poolside on a cruise at sea, a 67-year-old man is delirious and combative after being awoken from a nap by family. The patient is hyperthermic and eventually codes from hyperkalemia due to acute renal failure. The team must manage the patient as he declines and interact with family members and life partner who are in conflict regarding patient's goals of care. It is not clear who the decision maker should be: one of the patient's siblings or the non-married life partner. Cruise ship nurse and non-medical bystanders are available to assist.

2. TEACHING OBJECTIVES/DISCUSSION POINTS

Clinical and medical management

- Perform ABCDE and expose; obtain a full set of vital signs, identify and remove the dramamine patch
- Initiate appropriate work-up for an altered patient, including bedside testing-blood sugar and EKG
- Identify and manage hyperthermia including active cooling
- Identify and manage hyperkalemia

Communication and teamwork

- Determine patient capacity for making healthcare decisions
- Communication and conflict resolution with the family and life partner with conflicting opinions
- Code status determination
- Communication with physician at receiving medical facility

3. SUPPLIES

- Moulage make-up for sunburn
- Gray wig

■ Dramamine (dimenhydrinate) patch
■ Sunglasses, beach shirt, swim trunks, towel
■ Lounge chair
■ Cooling blankets, ice packs
■ Fan(s)
■ Water in buckets or spray bottles
■ Airway supplies: non-invasive and intubating supplies
■ IV tubing and fluids
■ Syringes marked with medications

4. MOULAGE

Mannequin with sunburn moulage, gray wig, beach shirt, sunglasses, swim trunks, overlying towel, motion sickness (i.e. Dramamine (dimenhydrinate)) patch behind ear.

5. IMAGES AND LABS

■ EKG3: sinus tachycardia, normal intervals, prominent T waves
■ The cruise ship can provide limited stat labs only. If requested, the following will be provided: bedside blood sugar, potassium, sodium, Hgb, hematocrit

6. ACTORS (CONFEDERATES) AND THEIR ROLES

■ Patient: a hybrid case where an actor plays the first part as the combative delirious patient but the case switches to simulator when the patient becomes unresponsive.
■ Nurse: the cruise ship nurse is neither helpful nor obstructive and relegates all decision making to the team.
■ Family members: various numbers of siblings of the patient, plus in-laws. Each member has a conflicting opinion of patient's wishes. They argue amongst themselves and try to draw the team into their conflicts, causing distraction and delays if not managed appropriately by team.
■ Life partner of patient: mostly helpful and cooperative with team, knows the most information about patient's medical history. Quiet and non-obstructive and tries to prevent family members from distracting the team.
■ Bystanders: willing to assist, but non-medical.
■ Consulting physician from nearby receiving medical facility (available by phone): neither obstructive nor helpful. Requests full report, questions management provided and demands team determines when patient is stable for transfer.

7. CRITICAL ACTIONS

■ Perform assessment of ABCDE
■ Identify and remove Dramamine patch
■ Initiate an altered mental status work-up, including bedside testing and broad work-up

■ Identify hyperthermia with CNS dysfunction, initiate aggressive cooling, manage shivering
■ Identify and treat hyperkalemia
■ Demonstrate appropriate communication skills with family and consulting physician

8. TIMELINE

Time 0

VS: none available

■ Summary of initial presentation: family states, "This is Uncle Joe, he's 67 years old, he's healthy as a horse. He fell asleep by the pool. We tried to wake him up but he was hard to wake up. He's been talking really funny since." Patient is combative and has not allowed IV access or vital sign assessment
■ History: family members offer limited information
■ Initial interventions: none
■ Physical exam
  ▶ General: opens eyes spontaneously, agitated, hot, dry
  ▶ HEENT: pupils 6 mm (dilated) equal/reactive, Dramamine patch behind ear
  ▶ Neck: supple
  ▶ Chest: CTA, normal
  ▶ Heart: normal sounds, regular
  ▶ Abdomen: normal sounds, soft, non-tender, non-distended
  ▶ Skin: no bruising, ecchymosis or signs of injury; hot, dry
  ▶ Extremities: no injuries noted
  ▶ Neuro: non-focal grossly, eyes opened, mumbling confused speech, moving all extremities awkwardly, not following commands

---

Critical actions
- Assess ABCs
- Obtain history
- Perform physical examination
- Identify and remove patch

Transition point 1: 2 minutes

VS: BP 90/40, HR 120, RR 24, O$_2$ Sat 95% RA, 43.5°C (only provided if team requests medical assistance and supplies from cruise ship nurse)

■ Changes in physical exam: no change from initial exam
■ If patient is calmed or sedated, the team will be allowed to continue with resuscitation
■ Labs: blood glucose 80
■ Imaging: if patient is placed on monitor, EKG will show sinus tachycardia, hyper-acute T waves
■ Cruise ship nurse offers assistance under the direction of the team. If medical supplies not requested at 2 minutes, the nurse should prompt the team

■ Family keeps asking questions "What is going on?" "WHAT are you doing to him?" and start using their cell phones to make calls to other family members
■ One family member develops chest pain (turns out to be sunburn to chest upon questioning/exam)

Critical actions
- Team must calm patient or sedate
- Request medical supplies from infirmary
- Obtain vitals signs
- Obtain IV access
- Place patient on monitor
- At least one team member should evaluate family member with chest pain

Transition point 2: 4 minutes(patient begins to worsen)

VS: BP 80/30, HR 70, RR 24, O_2 Sat 93% RA, 43.5°C

■ Changes in physical exam/condition:
  ▶ patient starts to make vomiting noises
  ▶ patient becomes less alert
■ If team initiates intubation without discussion with family, family becomes more angry and disruptive
■ If team hesitates to intubate, life partner gets upset and disruptive
■ Labs: limited stat labs. If requested, this can be provided to team at minute 4. potassium 6.5, sodium 133, Hgb 14, hematocrit 40
■ Imaging: EKG will show hyper-acute T waves, heart rate starts to slow with widening QRS
■ Family members obstructive towards intubation "our sister died of cancer on a ventilator; he wouldn't want that"
■ Life partner wants a full resuscitation, "he has no health problems, please just help him"

Critical actions
- Team must recognize deteriorating vitals and mental status
- Team must manage airway
- Request stat labs
- Team must initiate cooling
- Manage family members with conflicting needs
- Recognize change in rhythm
- Identify hyperkalemia

Transition point 3: 6 minutes (patient codes from hyperkalemia due to acute renal failure)

VS: cannot obtain BP, HR, or SPO

■ RR per bagging, 42.0°C, rhythm PEA
■ Changes in physical exam/patient condition

- ▶ patient unresponsive
- ▶ pulseless without spontaneous respirations
- ▓ Labs: repeat blood glucose and stat labs unchanged
- ▓ Nurse (confederate): should prompt, "I don't feel a pulse" if code not recognized by team
- ▓ If team manages code and hyperkalemia appropriately (calcium, epinephrine, insulin, D50) patient will regain pulse and vital signs
- ▓ If team does not manage appropriately patient will continue to deteriorate

Critical actions
- Recognize loss of pulses
- Initiate CPR
- ACLS protocol
- Treat hyperkalemia

Transition point 4: final actions (patient resuscitated adequately)

VS: BP 90/40, HR 120, RR as per vent or bagging, O_2 Sat 97%

- ▓ Changes in physical exam:
  - ▶ patient with spontaneous respirations
  - ▶ regular pulse
- ▓ If team has performed both active and passive cooling of the patient using a combination of cooling blanket, tepid water, ice bath, mist, fans, cold IV fluids, or foley/NG lavage the temperature will decrease to 40.3°C
- ▓ Consulting physician, either ICU cruise ship infirmary or hospital physician at nearest dock will accept report
- ▓ Family members and life partner request update
- ▓ Additional points:
  - ▶ consideration for management of shivering
  - ▶ consideration for drawing blood cultures and additional labs to be transferred with patient
  - ▶ consideration for initiating empiric antibiotics
- ▓ Disposition: to ICU infirmary aboard ship or request to dock for hospital transfer

Critical actions
- Continue aggressive cooling
- Continue treatment for hyperkalemia
- Discussion with family members
- Request for patient transfer
- Give report to consulting physician

9. STIMULI

- ▓ EKG3: sinus tachycardia, normal intervals, prominent T waves
- ▓ Labs:
  - ▶ bedside blood sugar 80
  - ▶ potassium 6.5

▶ sodium 133
▶ Hgb 14
▶ Hematocrit 40

10. BIBLIOGRAPHY

Riccardi A, Tasso F, Corti L, Panariello M, Lerza R. The emergency physician and the prompt management of severe hyperkalemia. *Intern Emerg Med* 2012; 7(Suppl 2):S131–s133.

Younggren B, Yao C. The evaluation and management of heat injuries in the emergency department. *Emerg Med Pract* 2006; 8:1–24.

Hypertensive emergency

Nikita K. Joshi and Yasuharu Okuda

1. SCENARIO OVERVIEW

A 55-year-old woman with history of end-stage renal disease (ESRD) on hemodialysis, with hypertension, diabetes and coronary artery disease found by neighbors after hearing the patient's dog barking in her apartment for over 2 hours. She is minimally responsive and lying on couch. Neighbor says he spoke to her the previous evening when she told him that she wasn't feeling well and has missed 4 days of dialysis. She arrives by ambulance. Pill bottles were found at beside and brought by EMS to show to the medical team: hydrochlorothiazide, amlodipine, Glucophage (metformin), aspirin. The medical work-up in the ED reveals renal failure, hyperkalemia and CHF. Patient goes into ventricular tachycardic arrest. Team should go through the AMS algorithm and must treat the elevated BP.

2. TEACHING OBJECTIVES/DISCUSSION POINTS

Clinical and medical management

- Diagnosis and management of AMS
- Importance of fingerstick glucose
- Recognition of hypertensive emergency
- Hyperkalemia management
- ACLS protocol
- Contraindications to succinylcholine during RSI

Communication and teamwork

- Obtaining history from all resources such as neighbor and EMS
- Working in an interdisciplinary team including EMS and nursing

3. SUPPLIES

- IV fluid
- Non-invasive airway supplies: nasal trumpet, NRB
- Intubation supplies: BVM, ETT, stylet, blade and handle, suction, back-up airway

■ Defibrillator and monitor with pads
■ Syringes for medication administration
■ Pill bottles

4. MOULAGE

Disheveled wig, dirty nightgown, left arm AV graft.

5. IMAGES AND LABS

■ CT1: normal head CT
■ EKG3: sinus tachycardia, normal intervals, prominent T waves
■ XR8: CHF
■ Labs: CBC, BMP, cardiac markers

6. ACTORS

■ Patient: mannequin.
■ Neighbor: comes with patient to the ED in the EMS vehicle, gives the team history of the missed dialysis, the barking dog and disheveled appearance of the patient.
■ Nurse: assists the team in following orders, administering medications, etc.
■ Lab technician (voice): provides results of critical values over the phone.
■ Renal consult resident (voice): discusses the case with the team, initially pushes back on the emergency dialysis, is concerned why the patient coded and ultimately agrees on the need for emergency dialysis.

7. CRITICAL ACTIONS

■ Recognize the critically ill medical patient
■ Identify a patient with altered mental status
■ Diagnose and treat hypertensive emergency
■ Institute medical management of hyperkalemia
■ Institute airway management of patient with hyperkalemia
■ Adhere to ACLS protocol

8. TIMELINE

Time 0

VS: BP 245/185, HR 85, RR 20, O_2 Sat 98% on 2 L, 37°C, fingerstick glucose 110 (given when asked for), EKG –sinus rhythm at 80 bpm

■ Summary of initial presentation: 55-year-old woman with history of ESRD on hemodialysis, with hypertension, diabetes, coronary artery disease found by neighbors because the dog was barking in her apartment for 2 hours. Has not been dialyzed in 4 days. Brought in by ambulance. Pill bottles found at bedside: hydrochlorothiazide, amlodipine, Glucophage, aspirin.

- Initial interventions: IV line placed in right AC, 20 gauge, without difficulty (AV graft in left arm)
- Physical exam
  ▶ General: minimally responsive, moans, disheveled, smells of urine, moderate respiratory distress
  ▶ HEENT: pupils 2 mm, equal/reactive
  ▶ Neck: supple
  ▶ Chest: diffuse crackles
  ▶ Heart: regular rate, no murmurs
  ▶ Abdomen: normal
  ▶ Skin: normal
  ▶ Extremities: AV graft with positive thrill
  ▶ Neuro: moves extremities symmetrically, does not follow commands
- Nurse: assist team in obtaining IV access, placing on a monitor, and initial exam
- Neighbor: provides history when asked by the team

Critical actions
- Obtaining IV access
- Obtaining fingerstick glucose
- Primary and secondary survey

Transition point 1: 1 minute

VS: BP 245/185, HR 85, RR 20, O_2 Sat 98% on 2 L, 37°C, EKG – sinus at 80

- Physical exam: unchanged
- Team orders head CT, EKG, labs
- Nurse asks: "What should we do with the BP doctor?"
- Team should consider: labetalol, nitroglycerin, nicardipine, nitroprusside, furosemide

Critical actions
- Address hypertensive emergency
- Order appropriate work-up for assessment of AMS

Transition point 2: 2 minutes

VS: BP 245/185, HR 85, RR 20, O_2 Sat 98% on 2 L, 37°C, EKG – sinus rhythm at 80

- Physical exam unchanged
- CT: calls for patient at time 2 minutes: images shown of normal head CT
- EKG shown: peaked T waves
- Critical Lab notification called: creatinine 9, potassium 7.2, bicarbonate 20
- Nurse asks team if they would like to administer any medications
- Renal consult: emergency dialysis will be arranged
- Team: should manage hyperkalemia: albuterol, calcium, bicarbonate, dextrose, insulin

> **Critical actions**
> - Interpretation of head CT, EKG, lab values
> - Medical management of hyperkalemia

Transition point 3: 4 minutes

VS:

- Treated BP: 190/140, HR 85, RR 30, Sat 92% on 100% NRB
- Not treated BP: 255/195, HR 85, RR 30, Sat 92% on 100% NRB
- Physical exam
    - General: now in respiratory distress, less responsive
    - Chest: tachypneic, decreasing O_2 saturation
    - Neuro: moves extremities symmetrically, does not follow commands
- Team should manage the airway using RSI, should not give succinylcholine
- Nurse points out the respiratory distress, obtains the medications and equipment that is requested

> **Critical actions**
> - Recognize deterioration of the patient
> - Secure a definitive airway
> - Avoid giving succinylcholine given the hyperkalemia

Transition point 4: 6 minutes

VS: BP 190/140 ventricular tachycardia, RR intubated, O_2 Sat 100% BVM

- Physical exam
    - General: intubated and paralyzed
    - Chest: bilateral breath sounds, improving O_2 saturation
    - Heart: pulseless
    - Neuro: paralyzed
- Cardiac arrest after intubation
- After two cycles of CPR per ACLS protocol and treatment of hyperkalemia, will have returned to spontaneous circulation
- Nurse performs all actions requested by the team

> **Critical actions**
> - Recognize rhythm change on the monitor
> - Initiate ACLS protocol
> - Treat hyperkalemia

Transition point 5: 7–8 minutes, final actions

VS: BP 190/140, HR 70, RR intubated, O_2 Sat 100% BVM

- Physical exam
    - Heart: strong regular pulse
- Page MICU for admission

Critical actions
- Stabilize post-arrest patient
- Arrange for final disposition

9. STIMULI

- CT1: normal head CT
- EKG3: sinus tachycardia, normal intervals, prominent T waves
- XR8: pulmonary edema
- Labs:
  - CBC: WBC 8, Hgb 8.9, hematocrit 28, platelets 180
  - BMP: sodium 132, potassium 7.2, chloride 103, bicarbonate 20, BUN 13, creatinine 9.0, glucose 200, calcium 9.3
  - cardiac markers: tropinin 0.05, creatine kinase 80

10. BIBLIOGRAPHY

Mallon WK, SM Keim, JM Shoenberger, RM Walls. Rocuronium vs. succinylcholine in the emergency department: a critical appraisal. *J Emerg Med* 2009; 37:183–188.

Neumar RW, CW Otto, MS Link et al. Part 8: adult advanced cardiovascular life support: 2010 American Heart Association guidelines for cardiopulmonary resuscitation and emergency cardiovascular care. *Circulation* 2010; 122:S729–S767.

Wolf JS, B Lo, RD Shih et al. Clinical policy: critical issues in the evaluation and management of adult patients in the emergency department with asymptomatic elevated blood pressure. *Ann Emerg Med* 2013; 62:59–68.

Adrenal insufficiency

Andrew Schmidt and Lisa Jacobson

1. SCENARIO OVERVIEW

A 70-year-old woman is found down by neighbors in her home, last seen normal 2 days prior. Only known history is hypertension and asthma. Upon arrival to ED, patient is altered, hypotensive, tachycardic and has evidence to suggest a hip fracture. Initial work-up shows lab values consistent with adrenal insufficiency, likely secondary to discontinuation of chronic steroids after suffering a femur fracture.

2. TEACHING OBJECTIVES/DISCUSSION POINTS

Clinical and medical management

- Initial resuscitation and stabilization of a hypotensive patient
- Proper initial work-up for an altered patient
- Detection of signs, symptoms and lab values consistent with adrenal insufficiency
- Proper medical management of hypotension associated with adrenal insufficiency

Communication and teamwork

- Early determination of team leader and member roles
- Early communication with EMS
- Efficient communication of patient condition and pertinent findings
- Communication with family upon their arrival
- Maintenance of environment conducive to critical thinking and effective communication

3. SUPPLIES

Mannequin with moulage as described below; airway supplies.

4. MOULAGE

Left leg shortened and externally rotated; areas of hyperpigmentation on skin.

5. IMAGES AND LABS

- EKG5: sinus bradycardia (HR, 50–60)
- XR2: normal female CXR
- CT3: normal head CT
- XR7: pelvis with left acetabular fracture

6. ACTORS (CONFEDERATES) AND THEIR ROLES

- Paramedic: provide known history as specified.
- Nurse: assists team with obtaining access, drawing blood for labs and providing communications as assigned by administrators.
- Family members (son and daughter): arrive at specified time and provide information as specified below.

7. CRITICAL ACTIONS

- Recognize undifferentiated hypotension and begin initial resuscitation with IV fluids
- Recognize AMS and declining clinical course and secure definitive airway
- Provide empiric antibiotics
- Treat hypoglycemia with IV dextrose
- Recognize findings consistent with adrenal insufficiency and treat with steroids

8. TIMELINE

Time 0

VS: BP 84/40, HR 52, RR 14, O_2 Sat 92% on 2 L NC, 35°C (rectal), EKG – sinus bradycardia

- Summary of initial presentation: 70-year-old woman found down in her home by neighbors, last seen normal 2 days previous. Neighbors state they think she has a long history of asthma and hypertension, but they are unsure of any medications she takes. EMS contacted family to let them know she was being taken to the hospital; they report that she does not drink or use drugs and that she is usually very active
- Physical exam
  - General: obtunded, not answering questioning
  - HEENT: dry mucus membranes, atraumatic
  - Neck: no JVD
  - Cardiac: bradycardic, regular pulse, otherwise normal
  - Lungs: normal
  - Abdomen: decreased bowel sounds, otherwise normal
  - Neuro: moans to painful stimuli without moving extremities, PERRL
  - Skin: hyperpigmentation
  - Extremities (if asked): left leg shortened and externally rotated; pulses and capillary refill are normal

■ Paramedic: provide information as detailed above
■ Labs: fingerstick glucose: 25

Critical actions
- Obtain detailed history from EMS
- Ask nurse to obtain IV access and begin 2 L normal saline IV fluid
- Obtain fingerstick glucose

Transition point 1: 2 minutes

VS:

■ ▶ BP if IV fluid given: remains the same despite fluid resuscitation
  ▶ BP if IV fluid not given: 70/46
  ▶ HR: remains the same despite fluid resuscitation
  ▶ O_2 Sat if patient intubated: 100%
  ▶ O_2 Sat if patient not intubated: 85% on NC or NRB
■ Changes in physical exam/condition
  ▶ Neuro: no change in mental status
  ▶ If more than 2 L IV fluid given, O_2 Sat drops 5% and rales on exam
■ Labs: fingerstick glucose 50 (if D50 given, if not it remains 25)
■ EKG: sinus bradycardia, otherwise normal
■ Imaging: none available

Critical actions
- Treat hypoglycemia with D50
- Evaluate and manage airway
- Initiate pressors
- Recheck fingerstick after initial D50

Transition point 2: 4 minutes

VS:

■ BP
  ▶ if no pressors: 66/30
  ▶ if norepinephrine: remains same as previous
  ▶ if dopamine: remains same as previous (90)
■ HR: remains the same despite fluid resuscitation
■ O_2 Sat:
  ▶ if patient intubated: 100%
  ▶ if patient not intubated: 80% on NC or NRB
■ Changes in physical exam/condition:
  ▶ if dose of steroids given, there is no immediate response
  ▶ if fingerstick glucose not rechecked after previous D50, patient will have seizure refractory to all treatment other than dextrose
  ▶ if patient not intubated at this point, she will vomit, aspirate, and arrest

■ Labs: fingerstick glucose 40 (whether or not D50 given)
■ Imaging: none available
■ Son, daughter (confederates) arrive: eager to see their mother, but are easily controlled if taken seriously
■ History from family: mother takes a pill every day for her asthma; she often takes extra, no other information/details known

Transition point 3: 6 minutes

VS: same as previous

■ Changes in physical exam/condition: if patient not intubated at this point, she will vomit, aspirate and arrest
■ Labs:
   ▶ fingerstick glucose 35 (whether or not D50 given)
   ▶ BMP: sodium 132, potassium 5.5, chloride 92, bicarbonate 19, BUN 30, creatinine 1.2
   ▶ CBC: WBC 11 (normal diff), all other values normal
   ▶ Urinalysis: ketones 50, otherwise normal
   ▶ Urine DOA: normal
   ▶ Serum alcohol: normal
   ▶ LFTs, cardiac enzymes, BNP, coagulation factors: normal
   ▶ Serum cortisol, ACTH, and thyroid function test: not available as stat results
   ▶ ABG/VBG: normal
   ▶ $ScVO_2$: 70
■ Lumbar puncture (LP): normal
■ Imaging:
   ▶ XR2: normal female CXR
   ▶ XR7: pelvis with left acetabular fracture
   ▶ CT3: normal head CT for age
   ▶ US1: normal RUSH (rapid US in shock examination); normal cardiac function, normal IVC, normal aorta, no free fluid in abdomen

Critical actions
- Start patient on dextrose drip
- Administer steroids

Transition point 4: 7 minutes

VS: BP

■ ▶ BP if patient on dextrose drip and steroids: 90/60
   ▶ BP if not on both dextrose and steroids: remains same as previous
   ▶ all other vital signs same as previous
■ Changes in physical exam/condition:
   ▶ if patient not started on dextrose drip after third dose of D50, patient will have seizure refractory to all treatment other than dextrose
   ▶ if orthopedics consulted before initiating treatment with dextrose, pressors and steroids, patient will decompensate

■ Labs: fingerstick glucose on dextrose drip 50, if not on dextrose drip 25
■ Son and daughter: anxious and needy if not appropriately involved and if not provided with updates

Critical actions
- Dextrose drip
- Steroids if not already
- Explain condition to family

Transition point 5: final actions

VS: same as previous, EKG – sinus bradycardia

■ Changes in physical exam/condition: if patient sent to OR, she will die on the table
■ Labs: fingerstick glucose if on dextrose drip 60, if not on dextrose drip 25
■ MICU and endocrine consultants: amenable to any plan by the team, but orthopedics consultation will request medical clearance by the ED team for surgery

Critical actions
- MICU consultation
- Orthopedic consultation
- Endocrinology consultation

9. STIMULI

■ EKG5: sinus bradycardia
■ XR2: normal female CXR
■ CT3: normal head CT
■ XR7: pelvis with left acetabular fracture

10. BIBLIOGRAPHY

Idrose AM. Adrenal insufficiency and adrenal crisis. In Tintinalli JE, Stapczynski JS, Cline DM et al. eds. *Tintinalli's Emergency Medicine: A Comprehensive Study Guide*, 7th edn. New York: McGraw-Hill, 2011, pp. 1453–1456.

Lapi F, Kezouh A, Suissa S, Ernst P. The use of inhaled corticosteroids and the risk of adrenal insufficiency. *Eur Respir J* 2012; 42:79–86.

Nieman LK. Clinical manifestations of adrenal insufficiency in adults. *UpToDate* 2013 (http://www.uptodate.com/contents/treatment-of-adrenal-insufficiency-in-adults, accessed 31 July 2014).

"Raving" altered mental status

Michael Falk

1. SCENARIO OVERVIEW

You are working in a community ER in the southwest when the volunteer EMS unit brings a man in his 20s from a campsite. The patient and his friends are on their way to "Burning Man" festival and stopped at the local campsite for a few days. They have been doing drugs (marijuana and MDMA [ecstasy]) and drinking. The patient was "tripping" and was climbing among the boulders and crevasses near the camp site and was gone for some time.

  After coming back to the bonfire and campsite, the patient started to complain of leg cramping and "twitching." Initially, his friends thought he was joking around but the pain increased over the next hour or so until he collapsed and "was like spasming, man!" EMS volunteer crew says he is arching his back and having strange movements but is talking to us and screaming in pain.

2. TEACHING OBJECTIVES/DISCUSSION POINTS

Clinical and medical management

- Differential for AMS in young person
- To look for other causes of AMS and *not* assume that it is the drugs
- Complete head-to-toe exam, in non-communicative patient
- RSI and securing airway in patient with AMS

Communication and teamwork

- Controlling situation with intoxicated patient and friends
- Ensuring that team members do complete exam on patient with AMS

3. SUPPLIES

"Party" clothes for the patient and friends to realistically simulate rave culture. Also lollipops, pacifiers and other "props" that are associated with "rave culture" and MDMA ingestion (stimulates tactile pleasure and that is part of reason for "pacifier" and other oral stimulants).

4. MOULAGE

This is a hybrid case, starts with an actor and then moves to a mannequin. Both will need to have scorpion's stings on either one or both feet. Since one sting is generally not sufficient for toxicity, at least two to three should be moulaged on the feet, which have open sandals. For transition from actor to simulator, patient starts to seize and this can be mimicked by the actor who also places "alka seltzer" tab in mouth (part of a tablet) which cause frothing/foaming at the mouth to help to stimulate airway compromise.

5. IMAGES AND LABS

None needed.

6. ACTORS (CONFEDERATES) AND THEIR ROLES

■ Patient: arrives and is having very serious and painful muscle spasms of the lower extremities. These are severely painful and the patient should be yelling and screaming in pain (caused by scorpion venom). Scorpion envenomation is associated with "roving-eye" movements and the actor will need to stimulate this as well to help with the classic presentation. Pain and severity of spasms should escalate to involve the entire body with arching of the back and screaming in pain despite team's interventions. These spasms should be 5–10 seconds long and should *not* resemble seizures to help the team with the diagnosis. After about 4–5 minutes, the patient should start foaming at the mouth and his O_2 saturation should drop, forcing them to move to the mannequin and to intubate the patient. To stimulate foaming of the mouth: a quarter of an an Alka-Seltzer tablet or similar product slipped into the mouth is activated by saliva; it causes a lot of foaming and bubbling but tastes terrible.
■ Nurse: should be helpful and not obstructive given the complexity of the case.
■ Ravers: at least three or four extras are needed to be his friends from the campsite who are all very "high" and intrusive at the beginning of the case. They will arrive about 1–2 minutes after the patient and should barge into the treatment area and be quite loud and happy. They are *not* violent or threatening but they are very high on MDMA: this means they like to get in close and they are very "touchy," because it stimulates tactile sensation; they should touch staff and each other. Despite being "high" they should be concerned and helpful and they can be easily "redirected" after an initial 1–2 minutes of chaos when they arrive. For example, one can provide information that the patient has no PMH, no allergies and can give the "story" of what happened.
■ EMS and security personnel: the EMS is a rural, volunteer unit and so is helpful but not really that well trained or with deep knowledge base. Security should be used to redirect intoxicated friends and help to calm the scene.

7. CRITICAL ACTIONS

■ Recognize and treat AMS
■ Recognize, treat and develop differential diagnosis for severe, painful muscle spasm

■ Manage airway in patient with AMS
■ Control extremely chaotic scene
■ Use all resources (i.e. intoxicated friends) to complete history

8. TIMELINE

Time 0

VS: BP 150/105, HR 130, RR 20, O_2 Sat 100% NRB, 39.2°C – sinus tachycardia

■ Summary of initial presentation: patient arrives c/o severe pain and muscle spasms. He is communicative and trying to talk with MDs and staff but can't complete sentences because of severe muscle spasms and pain (patient needs to have "escalating" muscle spasms over the next 3–5 minutes: get larger and larger and more painful)
■ Initial interventions: monitor, establish peripheral IV lines (preferably two large-bore catheters) and complete head-to-toe exam
■ Treat pain and muscle spasms, fentanyl is medication of choice
■ Physical exam
  ▶ General: patient is intoxicated but complains of severe pain and muscle spasms
  ▶ HEENT: both eyes appear to rove and do so together, lots of oral secretions and needs suctioning
  ▶ Neck: normal
  ▶ Chest: CTAB
  ▶ Heart: sinus tach
  ▶ Abdomen: soft, non-tender, non-distended, + bowel sounds
  ▶ Skin: hot to touch and has intermittent fasciculations, sting X2 (wearing sandals), on left foot but only if they check him while removing clothes
  ▶ Extremities: as above, only on initial exam if specifically sought
  ▶ Neuro: patient is clearly high but complains of pain and responds at times to questions; has fasciculations and "roving" eye movements and otherwise non-focal
■ EMS (confederate): arrives with patient and gives story

> **Critical actions**
> • Place on monitor
> • Establish IV access
> • Head-to-toe examination
> • Treat pain/spasms

Transition point 1: 2 minutes

VS: same as arrival

■ Patient should develop severe spasms and arching of back, screaming in pain despite treatments; worsening secretions
■ Friends arrive: they are all very intoxicated and intrusive and making comments about "this is what he did at camp," "he's having a bad trip," etc. They should be

very happy and *not* belligerent but are also "invading personal space" and very "touchy" with the staff. Should try to make scene very chaotic for couple of minutes and then let themselves be redirected and calm. One friend should give history, *if* the team calms the friends down in right fashion
■ Patient requires more pain medications and despite this has worsening muscle spasms and pain
■ Labs: none available
■ Imaging: none available

Critical actions
- Suction and maintain airway
- Control pain
- Control friends
- Get rest of history

Transition point 2: 4 minutes

VS: same with worsening O_2 saturation near 4 minutes

■ Patient has increasingly severe spasms, worsening secretions and should require more and more pain medication and/or muscle relaxant. Should develop worsening upper airway control due to secretions and medications and start frothing at the mouth around 4 minutes. This is the cue to switch to mannequin
■ Labs:
  ▶ CBC: mildly elevated WBC, otherwise normal
  ▶ CMP: increased potassium (5.4) with increased BUN/creatinine ratio (i.e. in early rhabdomyolysis from muscle spasms)
  ▶ CPK in the 1000s from muscle spasms
  ▶ PT/PTT/INR all normal
  ▶ ABG/VBG: pH 7.27, low PCO_2
  ▶ Urinalysis: large protein and blood
■ Imaging: none available
■ Friends: should be calmer and helpful and very concerned about friend's status
■ Team should recognize the abnormal lab values as rhabdomyolysis and initiate treatment: increase fluids and alkalinize IV fluid and urine

Critical actions
- Continue with pain/muscle relaxants
- Recognize impending airway issue
- Treat rhabdomyolysis

Transition point 3: 6 minutes

VS: BP 150/100, HR 102s, RR 16 but "gurgling" and frothing at mouth, O_2 Sat 93% on NRB and dropping

■ Patient is losing upper airway and needs RSI. Medications should be based on worries about increased potassium. Needs suction because of secretions

■ Needs to be paralyzed and sedated after airway established and confirm placement with *at* least two techniques

■ If not done, nurse should push team to treat rhabdomyolysis with fluids and alkalinization of fluid and urine

■ Labs: as above

■ Imaging: none

■ Friends: very worried and not obstructive

Critical actions
- RSI but "hyper-K"
- Manage rhabdomyolysis
- Paralysis and sedation

Transition point 4: final actions

VS: BP 130/84, HR 110, RR intubated 100% on O_2

■ Changes in physical exam: intubated

■ Consultants: accepting ICU MD should "push" for diagnosis of AMS/muscle spasms; if team cannot, ICU should provide

■ Friends: will need to explain to friends why he is being transferred and what happened

■ Disposition: transfer to ICU

Critical actions
- Arrange transfer
- Deal with friends
- Come up with definitive diagnosis

9. STIMULI

None.

10. BIBLIOGRAPHY

LoVecchio F. Scorpion stings in the United States and Mexico. *UpToDate*, 2012 (http://www.uptodate.com/contents/scorpion-stings-in-the-united-states-and-mexico, accessed 31 July 2014).

Quan D. North American poisonous bites and stings. *Crit Care Clin* 2012; 28:633–659.

Skolnik AB, Ewald MB. Pediatric scorpion envenomation in the United States: morbidity, mortality, and therapeutic innovations. *Pediatr Emerg Care* 2013; 29:98–103.

Two patients with altered mental status and cyanosis

Jacqueline A. Nemer and Jeanne A. Noble

1. SCENARIO OVERVIEW

Patient A is a 33-year-old man brought in by paramedics after collapsing in a fast food restaurant. He was staggering, confused, then collapsed. Upon ED arrival, **Patient A** is awake but altered. During **Patient A**'s primary survey, **Patient B** arrives and disrupts the ED team. He was with **Patient A** and he is also altered. Both patients become unstable with worsening cyanosis despite O_2 administration. Once methemoglobinemia is diagnosed and treatment is initiated, **Patient B** worsens, developing hemolytic anemia and reveals a PMH of glucose-6-phosphate dehydrogenase deficiency.

2. TEACHING OBJECTIVES/DISCUSSION POINTS

Clinical and medical management

■ Perform ABCDE with airway control and c-spine immobilization
■ Demonstrate a systematic approach and differential diagnoses to altered mental status and loss of consciousness, and order appropriate work-up
■ Diagnose methemoglobinemia and administer methylene blue
■ Recognize hemolytic anemia secondary to methylene blue and stop further treatment

Communication and teamwork

■ Effective professional interpersonal communication with patients, medic, ED staff, hospitalist and consultant
■ Verbalization of management priorities by team leader
■ Effective simultaneous management of two patients, with appropriate delegation of responsibilities to all available team members, including directing a team member to provide immediate assessment and care for **Patient B**

3. SUPPLIES

■ Non-invasive airway equipment, including O_2 and suction
■ Intubation equipment

- IV administration equipment
- Cervical collar for **Patient A**
- Confederate's clothing: attire for EMT, nurse, respiratory therapist and **Patient B**
- Chocolate-brown blood in ABG syringe and blood tubes
- Mock blue medication (methylene blue)
- Second gurney for **Patient B**

4. MOULAGE

Forehead abrasion on Simman, blue lip coloring suggestive of cyanosis (Simman and **Patient B**).

5. IMAGES AND LABS

- Bedside labs
- Serum labs
- EKG1: sinus tachycardia, normal intervals
- EKG6: sinus tachycardia, normal intervals
- XR1: normal male CXR
- XR3: normal male intubated CXR
- CT1: normal head CT

6. ACTORS (CONFEDERATES) AND THEIR ROLES

- **Patient B**: friend of **Patient A** who arrives altered and disruptive during the initiation of resuscitation of **Patient A**. If ignored, he becomes obstructive. If addressed directly, he is cooperative and provides additional history. He becomes confused, begins vomiting and collapses during intubation of **Patient A**.
- Medic: provides HPI for **Patient A**. **Patient B** provides irrelevant details after initial hand-off until dismissed by team.
- Nurse: performs IV access, bedside and serum blood tests as ordered. Provides prompting, as needed, to steer team toward correct diagnosis ("This ABG must be venous, it's so dark," "I can't get this pulse ox to work right, but the waveform looks good"). Resists taking **Patient A** to CT scanner with a low O_2 saturation.
- Respiratory therapist: available if requested. Asks for summary of patient presentation. Assists with airway supplies and airway management upon request.
- Poison control/toxicology consultant: available for telephone consultation, providing methylene blue indications and appropriate dosing if requested.
- ICU consultant: available for telephone consultation to prompt team to order methemoglobin level by CO-oximeter and/or lab assay.

7. CRITICAL ACTIONS

- Complete primary survey (ABCDE) with disability assessment prior to intubation
- Use c-spine stabilization with collar and in-line stabilization during intubation
- Understand non-invasive and invasive airway management

■ Institute appropriate work-up for altered mental status (including initial blood glucose, ABG and urine toxicology screen), with discovery and treatment of methemoglobinemia
■ Recognize hemolytic anemia with administration of methylene blue and termination of treatment

8. TIMELINE

Time 0

VS for **Patient A** on arrival: BP 125/80, HR 105, RR 26, O_2 Sat 71% on RA, 37.0°C, EKG – sinus tachycardia

■ Summary of initial presentation: **Patient A** is a 33-year-old man with cyanotic lips and altered, lying on gurney. Medic reports "Bystanders mostly provided the history, this patient isn't really talking. Per witnesses, this patient and another guy were at the restaurant. 15 minutes after they drank soft drinks, this patient started staggering and talking loudly, complaining of feeling lightheaded, he vomited, then he collapsed and fell to the ground. The other guy (**Patient B**) who was with him disappeared before we arrived"
■ Initial interventions: none pre-hospital
■ Physical exam
  ▶ General: fully dressed
  ▶ HEENT: cyanotic lips, +gag reflex, +abrasion on forehead
  ▶ Neck: midline trachea, no CS step-off, unable to assess CST due to AMS
  ▶ Chest: tachypnea, clear
  ▶ Heart: tachycardia, rate/rhythm regular, no muffling
  ▶ Abdomen: soft, normal bowel sounds, no bruising
  ▶ Rectal (if performed): normal tone, normal prostate position, no blood
  ▶ Skin: no rashes, no bruising, no lesions
  ▶ Neuro: arousable to tactile stimuli; GCS 11 (eyes 2, motor 5, voice 4, delayed, repetitive with nonsensical answers "Yes sir," "No drugs, I'm a lawyer")
■ Medic: gives the report, continues making useless comments until team redirects medic
■ Nurse: available to place IV line and draw labs upon request

Transition point 1: 2 minutes

VS for **Patient A**: BP 125/80, HR 105, RR 22, O_2 Sat 85% on NRB

■ **Patient B** stumbles into ED, as **Patient A**'s mental status declines to point of non-responsiveness
■ **Patient B**: yells "Where did you go? I went to the bathroom and when I came out you were gone." To the team, "I've got him now, guys, thanks, he'll rest it off and he'll be fine thanks"
  ▶ If disregarded, **Patient B** becomes obstructive. "I'm a lawyer, you don't have permission..."
  ▶ If addressed, **Patient B** remains cooperative and provides more history: "He has no PMH, we were just having fun, it's all cool," "no drugs, no alcohol," "nothing illegal, honest, we're lawyers in town for a personal injury convention"

■ Labs available (if ordered): glucose, ABG
■ Imaging: XR1
■ Nurse: when IV access is completed, "I've got the IV in" and holds up the lab tubes filled with brown blood. If needed, prompts "Are the blood gas results OK? I think it was venous, his blood was so dark." If no blood gas ordered, nurse prompts "I cannot get this pulse ox to read right, but the waveform looks OK"

Critical actions
- Primary survey
- Cervical spine stabilization

Transition point 2: 4 minutes

VS for **Patient A**: BP 125/80, HR 110, RR 10, O_2 Sat 85% NRB

■ **Patient A** is no longer responding to physical stimuli. If team does not prepare to intubate, **Patient A** develops loud, sonorous respirations and de-saturates to <70%
■ For intubation, team should provide c-spine immobilization, order RSI medication for suspected head injury, order post-intubation CXR and head CT
■ **Patient B**: starts to mumble, staggers and collapses face down during intubation of **Patient A**
■ Team members must assess **Patient B**: ABCDE and order IV access, O_2, monitor, blood sugar, EKG, suction

VS for **Patient B**: BP 120/72, HR 100, RR 22, O_2 Sat 91% RA; nurse reports VS if no second monitor

■ Summary of initial presentation: eyes closed, mumbled speech, answering questions, following commands
■ **Patient B** retches and belches during exam. "I thinking I'm going to puke," rolls over to his side
■ **Patient B**: PMH (if team asks):
   ▶ allergies to NSAIDs and aspirin, "I can't take a lot of medication, I can only use Vicodin or Percocet for pain"
   ▶ "some blood thing that runs in my family, I can't think of what it's called – can you name some?"
■ Labs available for **Patient A**: CBC, chem7, lactate
■ Labs available for **Patient B**: glucose
■ Imaging available for **Patient A**: XR3 (normal male intubated CXR)
■ Nurse: If CT ordered for **Patient** A, s/he insists "I am not comfortable taking this patient to CT until his pulse ox improves." Clinical decision must be discussed with nurse before proceeding
■ **Patient B**: collapses during intubation of **Patient A** (see above)
■ Respiratory therapist: arrives (if team requests), "I'm the respiratory therapist – who can give me report?"

Critical actions
- Intubation of **Patient A**

Transition point 3: 6 minutes

VS for **Patient A**: BP 132/68, HR 90, RR vent 85% with FIO_2 1.0 – sinus tachycardia

VS for **Patient B**: BP 120/72, HR 100, RR 22, O_2 Sat 91% RA – sinus tachycardia

- If ordered by team, CO-oximetry results are displayed for both patients
- Changes in physical exam/patient condition:
  - ▶ **Patient A** paralyzed and sedated
  - ▶ **Patient B** dry heaving: "pump my stomach, I need to get this stuff out. Pump his stomach too!"
  - ▶ If team questions, **Patient B** will disclose: "we bought a psychodelic herb off the Internet, it is totally legal – from a legit company. We mixed it in our sodas, he drank more than me"
- If CO-oximetry is *not* ordered yet, ICU MD calls:
  - ▶ "What's going on with your intubated patient? I'll get an ICU bed ready"
  - ▶ "What's the blood gas results? and CO-oximetry results?" Criticizes team if CO-oximetry not ordered
- Team must order:
  - ▶ methylene blue (1–2 mg/kg in a 1% saline solution IV over 3–5 minutes)
  - ▶ ± consult Poison Control for advice regarding dosing
- Labs available for **Patient B**: glucose
- Imaging available for **Patient A**: head CT
- ICU MD (confederate) as telephone consultant: if needed prompts team to consider methemoglobinemia as diagnosis
- Poison Control (confederate): if needed advises team regarding methylene blue indications and dosing

---

Critical actions
- Recognition and treatment of methemoglobinemia

Transition point 4: final actions

VS **for Patient A**: BP 132/68, HR 90, RR vent, O_2 Sat 85% with FiO_2 1.0

VS for **Patient B**: BP 100/72, HR 140, RR 30, O_2 Sat 84% RA

- While methylene blue is running into IV catheter, **Patient B** become markedly more SOB (due to hemolytic anemia), and complains of feeling lightheaded. "I can't breath, I think I'm gonna pass out!" "What are you giving me in this IV? "I can't take most meds because of my blood problem – G6DV or something"
- Team must order: stop methylene blue, ± consult hematology, exchange transfusion (or PRBCs), ± hyperbaric O_2
- Labs: CBC, LDH, haptoglobin
- Disposition: ICU MD gets report from team
- Case ends

Critical actions
- Recognition of hemolytic anemia due to methylene blue

9. STIMULI

Patient A

- ▓ EKG6: sinus tachycardia, normal intervals
- ▓ ABG on supplemental O_2
- ▓ XR1: normal male CXR (if ordered pre-intubation)
- ▓ XR3: normal male intubated CXR
- ▓ CT1 (normal head CT)
- ▓ Lab data:

pH	7.43
$PaCO_2$	35 mmHg
PaO_2	222 mmHg
O_2 Sat (FiO_2 0.21)	98%
BMP	
Lactate (normal 1.0–1.8 mmol/L)	1.9
Sodium	136 mEq/L
Potassium	4.0 mEq/L
Chloride	100 mEq/L
Bicarbonate	24 mEq/L
BUN	14 mg/dL
Creatinine	0.9 mg/dL
Glucose	90 mg/dL
CBC	
WBC (normal $3.8–10.8 \times 10^9$/L)	9
Hgb (normal 13.8–17.2 g/dL)	13.8
Hematocrit (normal 41–50%)	42
Platelets (normal $150–450 \times 10^9$/L)	338
Toxicology screen	
Ethanol	0
Acetaminophen	<1
Aspirin	<1
Urine DOA	Negative
CO-oximetry	
Oxyhemoglobin (normal 88–95%)	41
Carboxyhemoglobin (normal <1.5%)	1
Methemoglobin (normal <2%)	66.7

Patient B

- ▓ EKG1: sinus tachycardia
- ▓ ABG on supplemental O_2

pH	7.38
$PaCO_2$	39 mmHg
PaO_2	94 mmHg
O_2 Sat (FiO_2 0.21)	96%
BMP	
Lactate (normal 1.0–1.8 mmol/L)	2.3

CBC	
WBC (normal 3.8–10.8 × 10^9/L)	15
Hgb (normal 13.8–17.2 g/dL)	7.1
Hematocrit (normal 41–50%)	21
Platelets (normal 150–450 × 10^9/L)	234
Reticulocytes (normal 12–130 × 10^9/L)	190*
CO-oximetry	
Oxyhemoglobin (normal 88–95%)	55
Carboxyhemoglobin (normal <1.5%)	0.5
Methemoglobin (normal <2 %)	43.7
Other	
LDH (normal 105–333 U/L)	2005
Haptoglobin (normal 41–165 mg/dL)	<30

10. BIBLIOGRAPHY

Kusin S, J Tesar, B Hatten, et al. Severe methemoglobinemia and hemolytic anemia from aniline purchased as 2C-E (4-ethyl-2,5-dimethoxyphenethylamine), a recreational drug, on the Internet – Oregon, 2011. *MMWR* 2012; 61:85.

Prchal JT and XT Gregg. Red blood cell enzymopathies. In Hoffman R, Benz E, Sanford S et al. eds. *Hematology: Basic Principles and Practice*, 5th edn. Philadelphia, PA: Churchill Livingstone Elsevier, 2008, pp.561–576.

Rosen PJ, C Johnson, WG McGehee, E Beutler. Failure of methylene blue treatment in toxic methemoglobinemia. Association with glucose-6-phosphate dehydrogenase deficiency. *Ann Intern Med* 1971; 75:83.

SECTION 3

CARDIOPULMONARY

Severe asthma

Scott Goldberg and Yasuharu Okuda

1. SCENARIO OVERVIEW

A 29-year-old morbidly obese man is brought in by EMS with severe respiratory distress. He reports cough, sore throat and worsening asthma symptoms. His wife says he has been worsening over the past 5 days. Over the past several hours he has been using his pump every hour with minimal relief. About an hour ago he began to become confused and his wife called 911.

2. TEACHING OBJECTIVES/DISCUSSION POINTS

Clinical and medical management

- Appropriate differential diagnosis and initial interventions for critical respiratory distress
- Indications for, and utilization of, pharmacological agents for the management of severe asthma
- Appropriate management of the potentially difficult airway
- Post-intubation care focusing on ventilator management in severe asthma

Communication and teamwork

- De-escalate a worried spouse who may not understand the gravity of the clinical situation
- Work as a team to provide multiple interventions – in parallel – to a critically ill patient

3. SUPPLIES

None.

4. MOULAGE

Diaphoresis.

5. IMAGES AND LABS

XR3: normal male intubated CXR

EKG1: sinus tachycardia

6. ACTORS (CONFEDERATES) AND THEIR ROLES

- Wife: upset with husband that he did not seek medical attention early; generally disruptive until she is cleared from the scene.
- Nurse: generally helpful; may need to prompt team on ventilator alarms.
- MICU consult: non-obstructive, will take patient to ICU without argument.

7. CRITICAL ACTIONS

- Identify and appropriately manage a severe asthma exacerbation with respiratory distress
- Identify and manage the difficult airway using an appropriate strategy and techniques
- Render appropriate post-intubation care of the intubated patient
- Utilize an appropriate ventilator strategy for the intubated severe asthmatic

8. TIMELINE

Time 0

VS: BP 165/100, HR 130s, RR 30, O_2 Sat 90% NRB, 37.4°C – sinus tachycardia

- Summary of initial presentation: 29-year-old morbidly obese man brought in by EMS. Patient is tripoding, diaphoretic. He has received two albuterol nebulizer treatments en route. Paramedics have been unable to initiate IV access. He is refusing to keep facemask on
- PMH: asthma, has been intubated in the past; last admission 1 month ago
- Surgical history: none
- Social history: +smoker, denies drugs, denies alcohol
- Medication: albuterol, fluticasone
- Allergies: NKDA
- Initial exam:
  - ▶ General: agitated, diaphoretic, severe respiratory distress
  - ▶ Neck: supple
  - ▶ Chest: very poor air entry, no wheezes
  - ▶ Heart: regular rhythm, tachycardia
  - ▶ Abdomen: morbid obesity, soft, non-tender
  - ▶ Extremities: cyanotic
  - ▶ Skin: diaphoretic
  - ▶ Neuro: confused as to location
  - ▶ Glucose: 110
- Wife: arguing with husband, upset that he waited so long to call the ambulance
- Nurse: unable to obtain IV access for approximately 45 seconds

Critical actions
- Appropriate initial interventions for acute respiratory distress
- Attempt IV access, consider IO access
- Initial aggressive treatment for severe asthma including IM epinephrine
- De-escalate wife and attempt removal from scene

Transition point 1: 2 minutes (continued decompensation)

VS: BP 160/100, HR 130, RR 16, O_2 Sat 91% NRB

- Patient is progressively confused, minimally interactive, fatigued
- If all appropriate medications given
  - ▶ wheezes become apparent
  - ▶ patient will slowly decompensate
- If inadequate treatment: patient will precipitously decompensate
- Team should identify impending intubation and evaluate for potential difficult airway
- Labs: ABG (initial)

Critical actions
- Identify impending respiratory collapse
- Discuss an approach for airway management in the potentially difficult airway
- Consider an attempt at non-invasive ventilation

Transition point 2: 4 minutes (airway management)

VS: BP 160/100, HR 130, RR 8, O_2 Sat 88% NRB

- Patient is lethargic, minimally responsive
- If *anxiolytic or ketamine* is given with *BiPAP*: O_2 saturation will improve to 92–95% prior to intubation attempt
- If patient is paralyzed with *bagging* or placement of *EGA*: O_2 saturation will improve to 92–95% prior to intubation attempt
- If patient is paralyzed *without bagging* through apneic period:
  - ▶ O_2 saturation will precipitously drop to 50%
  - ▶ patient will begin to become bradycardic
- If airway is not managed:
  - ▶ patient will decompensate rapidly
  - ▶ patient will become bradycardic and suffer a cardiac arrest
- If difficult airway adjuncts are used: intubation proceeds successfully
- If no difficult airway adjuncts are used: unable to intubate patient, difficult to bag, desaturation

Critical actions
- Consideration of pretreatment prior to ETT placement
- Appropriate medication selection for induction and paralysis
- Appropriate utilization of difficult airway adjuncts

Transition point 3: final actions (post-intubation management and disposition)

If appropriate ventilation setting for permissive hypercapnea: BP 110/60, HR 110, O_2 Sat 94%

If ventilator settings are not adjusted: BP 140/90, HR 140, O_2 Sat 84%, alarm for high plateau pressure

■ Plateau pressure: 52
   ▶ will continue to alarm until disconnected from vent for manual exhalation
■ Labs: ABG (post-intubation)
■ Imaging: XR3 (normal male intubated CXR)
■ Nurse: may need to prompt team to recognize ventilator alarms
■ MICU: will take patient to ICU regardless of treatment

Critical actions
- Post-intubation management including ABG and CXR
- Analgesic and/or sedative drips
- Continue in-line albuterol nebulizers
- Ventilation management including low tidal volume, low or no PEEP, low respiratory rate, permissive hypercapnea
- Consider additional therapies including inhalation pharmacotherapy
- Appropriate disposition

9. STIMULI

■ XR3: normal male intubated CXR
■ EKG1: sinus tachycardia

10. BIBLIOGRAPHY

Brenner B, Corbridge T, Kazzi A. Intubation and mechanical ventilation of the asthmatic patient in respiratory failure. *J Emerg Med* 2009; 37(Suppl):S23–S34.

Cydulka RK. Acute asthma in adults. In Tintinalli JE, Kelen GD, Stapczynski JS, eds. *Emergency Medicine: A Comprehensive Study Guide*, 6th edn. New York: McGraw-Hill, 2004, Ch. 68.

Nowak RM, Tokarski G. Asthma. In Marx JA, Hockberger RS, Walls RM, eds. Rosen's Emergency Medicine: Concepts and Clinical Practice, 6th edn. Philadelphia, PA: Mosby-Elsevier, 2006, Ch. 72.

Rowe BH, Sevcik W, Villa-Roel C. Management of severe acute asthma in the emergency department. *Curr Opin Crit Care* 2011; 17:335–341.

Wood S, Winters ME. Care of the intubated emergency department patient. *J Emerg Med* 2011; 40:419–427.

High-altitude pulmonary edema with high-altitude cerebral edema

Michael Cassara

1. SCENARIO OVERVIEW

A 29-year-old man who is brought back to the base camp of a mountain climbing expedition with acute shortness of breath and altered mental status following a climb to higher elevation. The base camp is at 4500 m above sea level. The patient arrived at the base camp site yesterday after an ascent of 800 m. Yesterday evening the patient drank several "shots" of whiskey to celebrate his arrival. Late last night, the patient experienced a headache, nausea and vomiting, which he told others was likely from "partying a bit too much." In the morning, the patient went out with another climber and tried to ascend an additional 800–1000 m but could not as he began to complain of another severe headache, nausea and dizziness. He developed exertional dyspnea and breathlessness soon after heading out that did not resolve with rest. The other climber states that he had much difficulty persuading the patient to return to the base camp, as he was "coughing a lot and was having difficulty walking." The patient was also exhibiting signs of progressive confusion and attempted to take off his winter jacket (parka), gloves and hat several times during the return. The other climber was ultimately able to get the patient back to the base camp, which is where the patient care team meets him. The patient is confused, tachypneic, tachycardic and drowsy, with audible bilateral rhonchi and "rattling noises."

The base camp medical tent has the following capabilities:

- emergency blood glucose determination
- portable chest radiography
- portable low- and high-flow O_2 administration
- portable BiPAP
- portable mechanical ventilator
- 12-lead EKG
- portable cardioverter/defibrillator/transcutaneous cardiac pacer
- portable end-tidal capnography
- ABG (pH, PCO_2, PO_2, bicarbonate, O_2 Sat) with electrolytes and other serum analyses (sodium, potassium, calcium, glucose, Hgb, hematocrit, lactate)
- portable hyperbaric therapy.

Note: descent and medical evacuation is impossible because of severe inclement weather.

2. TEACHING OBJECTIVES/DISCUSSION POINTS

Clinical and medical management

- Define "high altitude," "very high altitude" and "extreme altitude"
- Describe the most common complications occurring with prolonged exposure to high-altitude environments, including, but not limited to:
  - ▶ acute mountain sickness
  - ▶ high-altitude pulmonary edema (HAPE)
  - ▶ high-altitude cerebral edema (HACE)
  - ▶ other environmental-related complications (e.g. hypothermia, cold-related soft tissue injuries, traumatic injuries)
- Demonstrate the appropriate initial management of a patient with acute HAPE
- Demonstrate the appropriate initial management of a patient with acute HACE

3. SUPPLIES

- Sleeping bag (to simulate a portable hyperbaric chamber)
- Equipment for O_2 administration (NRB mask, nebulizer, BVM, equipment for ETT placement advanced airway management)
- Winter parka and snowgear/clothes (for simulator and other climber [confederate])
- IV administration equipment
- "Mock" medications

4. MOULAGE

Young adult male mannequin, with cold, dry skin (ice packs or cooling blanket applied to external "skin"); "shivering" (tremor/seizure enabled) and make-up to give blue/gray lips and cyanotic nailbeds.

5. IMAGES AND LABS

- XR24: CXR with non-cardiogenic pulmonary edema
- Labs

6. ACTORS (CONFEDERATES) AND THEIR ROLES

- Patient: simulator.
- Other climber: mildly altered but helpful.
- Base camp nurse: helpful.
- Evacuation consultant: voice available by satellite telephone/base station radio; obstructive.

7. CRITICAL ACTIONS

- Administer high-flow supplemental O_2 (may require non-invasive or invasive ventilation)
- Request immediate descent (unable)

■ Initiate hyperbaric therapy (portable hyperbaric chamber available; initial recommendation: set chamber to 2 psi [13.8 kPa], which simulates a descent of approximately 2000 m)

■ Administer beta-adrenergic agonist (e.g. aerosolized salmeterol, initial dose 50 μg; or albuterol initial dose 2.5 mg (0.083%))

■ Administer dexamethasone (initial dose: 8 mg IV)

■ Administer carbonic anhydrase inhibitor (e.g. acetazolamide; initial dose: 250 mg PO; requires check of patient's allergies [sulfa])

■ Initiate rewarming strategies (passive and active such as warmed IV fluids, humidified air, heat packs and blankets)

Critical actions
- Administer high-flow O$_2$
- Request immediate descent
- Initiate rewarming strategies

8. TIMELINE

Time 0

VS: BP 140/90, HR 140, RR 36, O$_2$ Sat 85% RA, 33°C (91.4°F), EKG – sinus tachycardia with right heart strain pattern

■ Summary of initial presentation: 29-year-old man, with cold, dry skin, shivering, with blue lips and nailbeds (cyanosis), with acute shortness of breath and mental status change

■ No initial interventions at start of the case

■ Physical exam
  ▶ General: lethargy, diminished responsiveness, confusion, delayed cognition, slowed speech
  ▶ HEENT: frothy sputum (simulate with "mousse" at the oropharynx); no photophobia
  ▶ Neck: JVD, midline trachea, no meningismus
  ▶ Chest: tachypnea, rhonchi, audible wheezes; rapid, shallow breaths; persistent cough (hacking)
  ▶ Heart: tachycardia, rate and rhythm regular
  ▶ Abdomen: soft, without masses or tenderness, normal bowel sounds
  ▶ Rectal: normal tone, no blood
  ▶ Skin: no injuries; cold, dry skin; no rashes/track marks; cyanotic nailbeds
  ▶ Extremities: ataxia; uncoordinated movement of arms/legs; shivering
  ▶ Neuro: obtunded, lethargic and somnolent but arousable; localizes painful stimuli; no posturing; drowsy; shivering

■ Base camp nurse (confederate):
  ▶ assists with initial assessment and stabilization measures
  ▶ responds with serum glucose result ("fingerstick is 90 mg/dL") if bedside test is ordered
  ▶ is non-obstructive; helpful to team

■ Other climber (confederate):

   ▶ offers history of present illness, if asked

   ▶ describes the events of the preceding day, if asked

   ▶ is non-obstructive, helpful to team (may be altered at the discretion of session faculty)

   ▶ moves to perimeter of stage once delivery of key history is provided

■ Evacuation consultant (confederate), if called: is obstructive; unable to arrange for emergency descent or helicopter transport to base camp ("severe inclement weather has started, and evacuation is impossible")

Critical actions
- Administer high-flow O_2
- Request immediate descent
- Initiate rewarming strategies

Transition point 1: 1 minute

VS: BP 150/95, HR 140, RR 32, O_2 Sat 85–89%, 33°C (91.4°F)

■ IV access achieved after 1 minute (if ordered)

   ▶ serum for labs obtained and sent (if ordered)

   ▶ warmed IV fluids should be started

■ Response to supplemental O_2 after 1 minute (if ordered)

   ▶ increase O_2 Sat to maximum of 90–91%

   ▶ decrease RR to 30

■ Mental status, confusion, tachycardia, +/or O_2 Sat will worsen if delay in recognition of HAPE (failure to provide supplemental O_2) or HACE

■ Base camp nurse: assists team, uses "closed-loop" communication, remains non-obstructive

■ Evacuation consultant, if called: is obstructive; unable to arrange for emergency descent or helicopter transport to base camp ("severe inclement weather has started, and evacuation is impossible")

Transition point 2: 2 minutes

VS: BP 160/95, HR 140, RR 30, O_2 Sat 90–91%, 33°C (91.4°F)

■ Initial ABG results are available: pH, PCO_2, PO_2, bicarbonate, O_2 Sat

■ **At faculty discretion**: the need for ETT placement can be heightened or lessened. If the patient's condition is made so that ETT is required, then the team's ability to initiate hyperbaric therapy may be compromised. If the patient's condition is made so that ETT is not required (e.g. the patient's condition improves with non-invasive measures such as BiPAP and medical management), then the team should recognize the need for hyperbaric therapy and initiate it

■ Mental status, confusion, tachycardia, +/or O_2 Sat worsen if delay in recognition of HAPE (failure to provide supplemental O_2) or HACE

■ Team should consider rapid descent: not possible at this time (inclement weather)

■ Team should initiate rewarming strategies at this time
  ▶ warmed IV fluids (judiciously)
  ▶ humidified warmed O_2
  ▶ warming blanket
  ▶ heat packs to groin/axilla
■ Base camp nurse: responds with ABG result if test is ordered
■ Evacuation consultant, if called: is obstructive; unable to arrange for emergency descent or helicopter transport to base camp ("severe inclement weather has started, and evacuation is impossible")

Critical actions
- Administer beta-adrenergic agonist
- Administer dexamethasone
- Administer carbonic anhydrase inhibitor
- Initiate rewarming strategies
- Request immediate descent

Transition point 3: 4 minutes

VS: BP 170/95, HR 130, RR 30, O_2 Sat 91–93%, 34°C (93.2°F)

■ Response to rewarming strategies and supplemental O_2 administration (if ordered)
  ▶ decrease HR to 130
  ▶ increase temperature to 34°C
■ CXR results available at this time (if ordered): provide stimulus of XR24 (reveals non-cardiogenic pulmonary edema)
■ **At faculty discretion**: the need for ETT placement can be heightened or lessened. If the patient's condition is made so that ETT is required, then the team's ability to initiate hyperbaric therapy may be compromised. If the patient's condition is made so that ETT is not required (e.g. the patient's condition improves with non-invasive measures such as BiPAP and medical management), then the team should recognize the need for hyperbaric therapy and initiate it
■ Team should have considered rapid descent: not possible at this time (inclement weather)
■ Team should consider medication for HACE
  ▶ dexamethasone
  ▶ acetazolamide
  ▶ nifedipine (controversial)
  ▶ aerosolized beta-adrenergic agonist
  ▶ mannitol?
■ Mental status, confusion worsen if delay in recognition of HACE
■ Team should have initiated rewarming strategies by this time
  ▶ warmed IV fluids
  ▶ humidified warmed O_2
  ▶ warming blanket
  ▶ heat packs to groin/axilla
■ Base camp nurse: facilitates CXR and provides stimulus

■ Evacuation consultant, if called: is obstructive; unable to arrange for emergency descent or helicopter transport to base camp ("severe inclement weather has started, and evacuation is impossible")

Critical actions
- Administer beta-adrenergic agonist
- Administer dexamethasone
- Administer carbonic anhydrase inhibitor
- Initiate hyperbaric therapy

Transition point 4: 5 minutes

VS: BP 170/95, HR 120, RR 28–30, O₂ Sat 93–95%, 34°C (93.2°F)

■ EKG obtained/provided at this time (if ordered): sinus tachycardia, right heart strain pattern indicating pulmonary hypertension
■ Labs available (if ordered): additional serum analyses (electrolytes, hemoglobin, hematocrit)
■ Team should recognize HACE and order medications by this time: *if* medications administered, improve BP and do not worsen mental status or confusion
■ Mental status: confusion worsen if delay in recognition of HACE: at faculty discretion, seizure/coma/herniation will develop
■ Team should have initiated initial rewarming strategies by this time
■ Team should initiate hyperbaric therapy at this time: can provide sleeping bag as prop for portable hyperbaric chamber
■ Base camp nurse:
  ▶ facilitates tests that are ordered and provides stimulus, as appropriate
  ▶ suggests need for hyperbaric therapy (provides sleeping bag as prop for portable hyperbaric chamber)

Critical actions
- Request immediate descent

Transition point 5: final actions

VS: BP 160/70, HR 110, RR 22–24, O₂ Sat 95%, 37°C (98.6°F)

■ EKG should have been obtained/provided by this time
■ Additional serum analyses (electrolytes, hemoglobin, hematocrit) should have been obtained/provided by this time
■ Mental status, confusion should be improving if HACE has been recognized
■ Team should have initiated initial rewarming strategies by this time
■ Base camp nurse:
  ▶ notes "weather has miraculously improved"
  ▶ suggests consultation one more time with evacuation consultant
■ Evacuation consultant, if called: is non-obstructive; able to arrange for emergency descent or helicopter transport to base camp ("there has been a brief respite from the severe inclement weather and we believe we have a narrow window of opportunity to begin evacuation")

9. STIMULI

■ XR24: CXR with non-cardiogenic pulmonary edema
■ Labs

Test	Reference range/normal	Result
BMP		
Sodium	135–145 mEq/L	149
Potassium	3.5–5 mEq/L	4.0
Chloride	95–105 mEq/L	100
Bicarbonate	22–28 mEq/L	22
BUN	8–18 mg/dL	28
Creatinine	0.6–1.2 mg/dL	0.9
Glucose	70–110 mg/dL	100
WBC	3200–9800/mm^3	13,700/mm^3
Hgb	12.6–17.2 g/dL (male)	14
Hematocrit	39–49% (male)	44
Platelets	150 000–450 000/mm^3	450
pH	7.35–7.45	7.48
PaCO$_2$	40 mmHg	25
PaO$_2$	100 mmHg (FiO$_2$ 0.21)	46
Bicarbonate	22–28 mEq/L	22
O$_2$ Sat (FiO$_2$ 0.21)	97–100%	84
Lactate	<2 mmol/L	3.9

10. BIBLIOGRAPHY

Fiore DC, Hall S, Shoja P. Altitude illness: risk factors, prevention, presentation, and treatment. *Am Fam Physician* 2010; 82:1103–1110.

Gallagher SA, Hackett PH. High-altitude illness. *Emerg Med Clin North Am* 2004; 22:329–355.

Hackett PHH, Roach RC. High-altitude illness. *N Engl J Med* 2001; 345:107–114.

Hackett PH, Roach RC. High-altitude medicine and physiology. In Auerbach PS, ed. *Wilderness Medicine*, 6th edn. Philadelphia, PA: Mosby-Elsevier, 2012, pp. 2–33.

Hackett PH, Shlim DR. Altitude illness. Atlanta, GA: Centers for Disease Control and Prevention, 2013 (http://wwwnc.cdc.gov/travel/yellowbook/2014/chapter-2-the-pre-travel-consultation/altitude-illness, accessed 31 July 2014).

Wedmore I, Laselle BT. Altitude illness: strategies in prevention, identification, and treatment. *Emerg Med Pract* 2007; 9:1–24.

SCUBA: air embolism

Jason Wagner, Christopher Sampson and Brian Bausano

1. SCENARIO OVERVIEW

A SCUBA diver who ascended too quickly and has decompression illness complicated by acute MI. Friends are not sure if he ascended because of chest pain or not.

2. TEACHING OBJECTIVES/DISCUSSION POINTS

Clinical and medical management

- Expanded differential diagnosis for cerebrovascular accidents (CVAs)
- Acute management decisions for combined cardiovascular and cerebrovascular events
- Benefits in using supplemental O_2 as temporizing measure in treatment of air emboli
- In decompression illness *must **dive*** the patient

Communication and teamwork

- Good leadership directing the team
- Coordination to address both the cardiovascular and cerebrovascular events
- Logistics of coordinating with multiple specialties (cardiology, neurology, hyperbarics)

3. SUPPLIES

Male patient with swim trunks, wet suit or other appropriate swimming gear.

4. MOULAGE

None.

5. IMAGES AND LABS

- EKG7: STEMI
- CT13: normal head CT, multiple slices
- Fingerstick glucose 123 (verbal report)

6. ACTORS (CONFEDERATES) AND THEIR ROLES

- Patient: in swim wear.
- Nurse: facilitates and helps team as asked.
- Consultant cardiologist: reluctant to catheterize with neurological complaints.
- Consultant neurologist: reluctant to take patient with MI on EKG.
- Consultant hyperbarics: happy to help and can have dive chamber ready at end of case.
- Friend: cooperative and can help with history.

7. CRITICAL ACTIONS

- Obtain EKG and acknowledge acute MI
- Obtain CT head and acknowledge normal head CT
- Provide supplemental O_2
- Get patient to dive chamber

8. TIMELINE

Time 0

VS:– **sinus tachycardia at 88**

- Summary of initial presentation: 55-year-old male with right-sided facial droop, slurred speech, difficult to gather history, both confused and hard to understand. Presents as a "Code stroke" activated by triage nurse and brought back to room
- Physical exam
  - ▶ General: anxious, confused, hard to understand, appears stated age; in swim trunks, wet
  - ▶ HEENT: face indented by goggles, right facial droop, PERRL; patient becomes more anxious (but hard to understand) when realizes cannot see well
  - ▶ Chest: CTAB
  - ▶ Heart: regular rate and rhythm
  - ▶ Abdomen: soft, non-tender, non-distended
  - ▶ Skin: wet, no wounds
  - ▶ Extremities: normal, holding on to goggles
  - ▶ Neuro: right facial droop, slurred speech, moves all extremities, does not quite understand requests to test coordination, does not track well
- Nurse: struggles to get monitor leads on secondary to wet skin

---

Critical actions
- IV access
- Oxygen
- Monitor: must dry patient to get leads to stick

Transition point 1: 2 minutes

VS: BP 185/90, HR 88, RR 16, O_2 Sat 99% on RA, 37.0°C

- Patient gesturing toward chest, attempting to vocalize chest pain, very frustrated
- If placed on NRB (at any time in progression) some neurological deficits will improve

■ EKG: inferior MI
■ Nurse: "I think he's saying my chest hurts"

Critical actions
- EKG
- Call out to cardiology

Transition point 2: 4 minutes

VS: BP 185/90, HR 88, RR 16, O_2 Sat 99% RA, 37.0°C

■ Imaging: CT ready for patient
■ Friend/s available for more information
  ▶ no PMH
  ▶ can relate details of dive and rapid ascent
■ Stroke team (on phone) if called: request full exam, nervous due to MI
■ Consultant cardiologist (on phone) if called: nervous due to stroke symptoms

Critical actions
- CT head
- Call out to stroke team (or discuss treatment for CVA)

Transition point 3: 6 minutes

VS: BP 185/90, HR 88, RR 16, O_2 Sat 99% RA, 37.0°C

■ CT head: normal
■ Nurse: if asked to setup lytics can question whether this is for MI or CVA
■ Consultant cardiologist:
  ▶ reluctant to take to catherization with neurological symptoms
  ▶ keeps circling back to EKG being likely related to diving
  ▶ offers no solid help on air embolism
■ Consultant neurologist:
  ▶ concerned about cardiac symptoms
  ▶ discourages lytics
  ▶ will not provide useful information on air embolism if asked
■ Additional information: consultants and/or friends can suggest diving or relate experiences about dive chamber/air emboli if team is struggling

Critical actions
- Recognize need to dive
- Set up hyperbaric chamber

Transition point 4: final actions

VS: BP 185/90, HR 88, RR 16, O_2 Sat 99% RA, 37.0°C

■ Dive chamber ready

Critical actions
- Send to hyperbaric chamber

9. STIMULI

EKG7: STEMI
CT13: normal head CT, multiple slices

10. BIBLIOGRAPHY

Delaney MC, Bowe CT, Higgins GL. Acute stroke from air embolism after leg sclerotherapy. *West J Emerg Med* 2010; 11:397.

Prasad A, Banerjee S, Brilaks ES. Hemodynamic consequences of massive coronary air embolism. *Ciculation* 2007; 115:e51–e53.

Left ventricular assist device

Neal Aaron and Lisa Jacobson

1. SCENARIO OVERVIEW

A 62-year-old man with a history of stage 4 CHF has had a left ventricular assist device (LVAD) for 4 months and presents to community ED because his pump is beeping. His family is vacationing from another state. They decided to take a vacation because Dad has been feeling so well lately. They were out golfing when his pump started beeping.

2. TEACHING OBJECTIVES/DISCUSSION POINTS

Clinical and medical management

- Highlight that power (plug/batteries) is a necessity
- Identify life-threatening complications affecting patients with LVAD
- Recognize impediments to normal patient assessment and work arounds
- Learn appropriate management of dysrhythmia in LVAD

3. SUPPLIES

- LVAD power pack, plug and batteries
- Defibrillator
- Manual BP cuff

4. MOULAGE

Mannequin with LVAD.

5. IMAGES AND LABS

- EKG13: ventricular tachycardia
- XR27: left ventricular assist device

6. ACTORS (CONFEDERATES) AND THEIR ROLES

■ Patient: answer questions appropriately.
■ Nurse: assists team.
■ Consult: unavailable.
■ Wife: knows a lot about the machine and his history if appropriately asked.
■ Adult children of patient: very worried.

7. CRITICAL ACTIONS

■ Recognize power (plug/batteries) are a necessity
■ Institute appropriate management of dysrhythmia in LVAD
■ Recognize that compressions are contraindicated in LVAD
■ Recognize and implement appropriate actions to assess cardiovascular function in LVAD
■ Recognize the need to contact LVAD center and transfer patient

8. TIMELINE

Time 0

VS: BP unable to obtain, HR 100, RR 14, O_2 Sat 94% RA, 37.0°C, EKG – left bundle branch block in 100s

■ Summary of initial presentation: middle-aged man, in no acute distress, able to answer questions; LVAD alarm is beeping
■ Initial interventions: IV lines placed by EMS, prehospital 12-lead, etc.
■ Physical exam
  ▶ General: well nourished, well developed
  ▶ HEENT: normal
  ▶ Cardiovascular: rolling thrill sound, no obvious S1S2; no palpable pulse
  ▶ Respiratory: difficult to hear over pump sound
  ▶ Abdomen: pump palpable, no tenderness, wearing holster
  ▶ Extremities: no edema
  ▶ Neuro: normal

Transition point 1: 1 minute

VS: BP *nurse still cannot obtain*, HR 100, RR 14, O_2 Sat 94% RA

■ No changes in physical exam
■ IV access easily obtained if requested
■ Beeping sound permeates throughout ED; others start (mildly) complaining about noise
■ Labs: none available
■ Imaging: none available
■ Wife: complains mildly about noise from beeping LVAD

Transition point 2: 2 minutes

VS: no change

- Changes in physical exam/condition: none
- Family members firmly advocate that they know what to do, pressing random buttons on the pump, wiping Dad's brow, wondering where that phone number they're supposed to call is located. They note that they didn't bring an extra battery (if asked) but could go get one from the hotel
- If the LVAD is plugged in, beeping stops
- Labs: none available
- Imaging: CXR
- Adult family and wife: push buttons on pump, ask distracting questions and become increasingly louder

Critical actions
- Recognize need for power source or batteries

Transition point 3: 3 minutes

VS: BP unable to obtain HR 160, RR 18, O_2 Sat 94% RA – ventricular tachycardia in 160s

- Unable to feel pulse or obtain blood pressure
- EKG rhythm changes to ventricular tachycardia (can be managed)
  - ▶ with amiodarone or lidocaine and a fluid bolus: a different beep permeates the ED
- Patient is mentating normally
- Team may decide to measure Doppler flow with sonography, place arterial line (shows continuous pressure, no pulsatile flow), or measure $ETCO_2$
- Family: inquire as to new beeping, become annoyed that the beeping has not stopped

Critical actions
- Appropriate management of dysrhythmia in LVAD
- Recognize work around to assess cardiovascular status

Transition point 4: final actions

VS: unchanged (per management above)

- Patient is now more diaphoretic, confused and then rapidly non-responsive, despite initiation of drips of amiodarone or lidocaine (more so if no medications are started)
- If arterial line is placed: no pulse seen, $ETCO_2$ drops from 40s to 20s
- Defibrillation suggested: *no* compressions; two shocks acceptable, with medications in between
- If compressions are initiated and family members remain in room they will loudly admonish the providers that he's not supposed to receive CPR. If family is not in

room, the nurse will comment that she is certain she remembers learning compressions were contraindicated in patients with an LVAD
- ■ The phone number for the nearest LVAD center becomes available
- ■ Family: extremely upset, panicky, distraught and intrusive; they comment on compressions as above
- ■ Nurse: assist with tasks; comment that compressions are contraindicated
- ■ Disposition: transfer to LVAD center

Critical actions
- • Recognize shocks are appropriate without compressions
- • Transfer patient

9. STIMULI

- ■ EKG13: wide QRS
- ■ XR27: left ventricular assist device

10. BIBLIOGRAPHY

Cesario, DA, Saxon LA, Cao MK, Bowdish M, Cunningham M. Ventricular tachycardia in the era of ventricular assist devices. *J Cardiovasc Electrophysiol.* 2011;22(3):359–363.

Mechanical Circulatory Support Organization. *EMS Guide*, 2012 (http://www.mylvad.com/assets/ems_docs/00003528-2012-field-guide.pdf, accessed 31 July 2014).

Weingart S. Left ventricular assist devices (LVADS)." *EMCrit Blog* 2013 (http://emcrit.org/wee/left-ventricular-assist-devices-lvads/, accessed 31 July 2014).

CASE 15

Aortic dissection mimicking ST segment elevation myocardial infarction

Jason Wagner, Christopher Sampson and Brian Bausano

1. SCENARIO OVERVIEW

A 42-year-old man arrives by personal transport from restaurant after sudden onset of chest pain. EKG shows ST segment elevation myocardial infarction (STEMI) but patient has aortic dissection. CXR shows mediastinal widening. The team will need to diagnose aortic dissection and appropriately treat. Confrontation is created when the patient's neighbor who is a cardiologist arrives and demands lytics due to the cath lab being closed for floor waxing. The patient's spouse sides with cardiologist forcing the team to skillfully explain their reasoning.

2. TEACHING OBJECTIVES/DISCUSSION POINTS

Clinical and medical management

■ Proper differentiation between STEMI and aortic dissection
■ Importance of CXR prior to administration of lytics in patients with chest pain
■ Differentiate type A from type B aortic dissection
■ Proper treatment of aortic dissection

Communication and teamwork

■ Rapid coordinated communication and teamwork to properly differentiate STEMI from aortic dissection
■ Communication skills to explain difficult differentiating concepts with families and patients
■ Communication skills and professionalism to go against the trusted friend and cardiologist

3. SUPPLIES

None.

4. MOULAGE

None.

5. IMAGES AND LABS

- XR9: CXR with wide mediastinum
- EKG11: STEMI
- US2: cardiac US
- CT4: type A aortic dissection

6. ACTORS (CONFEDERATES) AND THEIR ROLES

- Patient: man in forties; the case could run with only an actor, only a mannequin or may need to run as hybrid if the actor has cardiac arrest from mismanagement requiring code resuscitation on mannequin.
- Nurse: facilitates care.
- Consult: cardiologist who is neighbor and friend and is demanding and pushy. Focused on STEMI and demands lytics while being indignant that "This hospital's Cath Lab is closed!" Moderate level of obstructionism based on how well team is performing.
- Wife: concerned about husband's welfare and sides with cardiologist until careful explanation given as to why lytics are not the correct action.
- Consult cardiothoracic surgeon: cooperative and willing to come in as soon as diagnosis is made. Delays arrival to force team to manage blood pressure. May suggest that BP be managed if team is not moving in that direction.

7. CRITICAL ACTIONS

- Diagnose STEMI on EKG
- Obtain and properly interpret CXR as widened mediastinum
- Obtain and properly interpret CT chest as type A aortic dissection
- Contact cardiothoracic surgery
- Control BP

8. TIMELINE

Time 0

VS: BP 170/90, HR 95, RR 20, O_2 Sat 99% NC, 37.2°C, EKG – sinus tachycardia with inferior ST elevations

- Summary of initial presentation: patient is uncomfortable in moderate distress, anxious and diaphoretic; cannot sit still or get comfortable; ill-appearing. Complains of chest pain over 2 hours, started while showering for work. Pain is substernal and sharp. Mild shortness of breath. No nausea or vomiting. No abdominal pain. No aggravating or alleviating factors. If asked specifically he admits that pain radiates to back
- Physical exam
  - General: moderate distress, anxious, awake, alert and orientated to date, place and person, well nourished, well developed
  - HEENT: within normal limits

> ▶ Heart: tachycardia, regular rhythm, no m/r/g
> ▶ Chest: lungs clear, no reproducible chest pain
> ▶ Abdomen: soft, non-tender, non-distended, normal bowel sounds, no hepatosplenomegaly
> ▶ Extremities: no cyanosis/clubbing/edema, peripheral pulses 2+ and symmetric throughout
> ▶ Psych: normal mood, appropriate behavior, mildly anxious, normal affect
> ▶ Neuro: non-focal, no deficits noted

■ Cardiologist friend: states that he thinks patient is having STEMI and demands EKG if team is not obtaining

Critical actions
- Obtain EKG
- Obtain IV access
- Obtain chest pain Labs

Transition point 1: 2 minutes

VS: BP 170/90, HR 95, RR 20, O_2 Sat 99% NC, 37.2°C

■ Changes in physical exam: none
■ If team is not moving toward EKG then patient claims of increasing chest pain
■ If team is moving quickly, ramp up cardiologist and wife's interference
■ Labs: none available
■ Imaging: EKG11 showing STEMI
■ Wife: worried and fretting
■ Cardiologist friend: remain demanding

Critical actions
- Interpret EKG as STEMI
- Order and obtain CXR
- Decision of cath lab vs. lytics
- Interpret CXR

Transition point 2: 5 minutes

■ VS: BP 170/90, HR 95, RR 20, O_2 Sat 99% NC, 37.2°C
■ Patient complains of increasing cardiac pain if team is not working towards STEMI
■ Imaging: XR9 (CXR with wide mediastinum)
■ Cardiologist friend: demands that lytics be given as "Time is muscle"
■ Team should be considering dissection in differential. If they are not then patient may complain of chest pain radiating to back

Critical actions
- Obtain chest CT
- Interpret CT
- Call CT surgery
- Control BP

Transition point 3: 7 minutes

VS: BP 200/90, HR 95, RR 20, O_2 Sat 99% NC, 37.2°C

■ If lytics given patient has cardiac arrest secondary to pericardial tamponade. This can be reversed by CPR, pericardiocentesis, and cardiothoracic surgery taking patient to OR
■ Labs: none available
■ Imaging: CT chest, cardiac US
■ Cardiologist friend: continues to demand lytics until it is tactfully explained that patient appears to have aortic dissection
■ Wife: continues to side with cardiologist until the situation is explained to her in layman's terms
■ Preferred BP control should be done with beta-blockers

> **Critical actions**
> • Control BP: beta-blockers, pain control
> • Cardiothoracic surgery to bedside

Transition point 4: final actions

VS:

■ ▶ if BP controlled: BP 110/60, HR 70, RR 16, O_2 Sat 99% NC, 37.2°C
  ▶ if BP *not* controlled: BP 220/102, HR 95, RR 20, O_2 Sat 99% NC, 37.2°C
■ Changes in physical exam: worsening pain, loss of pulse in right arm
■ Cardiothoracic surgeon: takes patient to OR and terminates case
■ Additional points: consider type and cross of blood products
■ Disposition: to OR

9. STIMULI

■ XR9: CXR with wide mediastinum
■ EKG11: STEMI
■ US2: cardiac US
■ CT4: type A aortic dissection

10. BIBLIOGRAPHY

Cook J, Aeschlimann S, Fuh A, et al. Aortic dissection presenting as concomitant stroke and STEMI. *J Hum Hypertens* 2007; 21:818–21.

Patel PD, Arora RR. Pathophysiology, diagnosis, and management of aortic dissection. *Ther Adv Cardiovasc Dis* 2008; 2:439–68.

Spittell PC, Spittell JA, Jr., Joyce JW, et al. Clinical features and differential diagnosis of aortic dissection: experience with 236 cases (1980 through 1990). *Mayo Clin Proc* 1993; 68:642–51.

Procedural sedation gone wrong in patient with upper gastrointestinal hemorrhage

Christopher Sampson and Jason Wagner

1. SCENARIO OVERVIEW

A 45-year-old man with history of hepatitis C and esophageal varices presented to ED with hematemesis. On team's arrival in room, patient is undergoing esophagogastro-duodenoscopy (EGD) with propofol sedation all coordinated by the GI MD. Nurse calls to team saying she is concerned patient is oversedated due to decreased responsiveness and hypotension. Immediately GI MD will note acute hemorrhage occurring at varices. Increasing tachycardia and hypotension result. GI MD will refuse to stop procedure – "give me one more minute, almost there." Team needs to force MD to stop procedure, manage airway with hematemesis and control hemorrhage. Blood products or Blakemore may be used.

2. TEACHING OBJECTIVES/DISCUSSION POINTS

Clinical and medical management

- Objective 1: recognize need to stop procedural sedation when patient unstable
  - demand obstructive physician stop procedure
  - turn off propofol infusion
  - treat hypotension
- Objective 2: know appropriate treatment of upper GI hemorrhage
  - IV fluids
  - red blood cell transfusion
  - massive transfusion protocol when initial efforts fail

Communication and teamwork

- Objective 1: team needs to initially force GI MD to stop procedure
- Objective 2: team communication with nurse confederate

3. SUPPLIES

Simulator, stretcher, replica endoscopic device, Blakemore tube.

4. MOULAGE

None.

5. IMAGES AND LABS

Video of EGD with hemorrhage (not provided).

6. ACTORS (CONFEDERATES) AND THEIR ROLES

- GI MD: refuses to stop procedure despite patient becoming critically ill.
- Nurse: assists team.

7. CRITICAL ACTIONS

- Stop GI from continuing with sedation and procedure
- Stop procedural sedation medications
- Treat hypotension with IV fluid and PRBCs
- Order massive transfusion protocol
- Manage airway
- Place Blakemore tube

8. TIMELINE

Time 0

VS: BP 80/40, HR 130, HR 8, O_2 Sat 88%, 37°C, EKG – sinus tachycardia

- Summary of initial presentation: 45-year-old man undergoing EGD with propofol sedation who is hypotensive and not responsive
- Initial interventions:
  - 18-gauge peripheral IV line place prior to start of scenario
  - O_2 via nasal canula
- Physical exam
  - General: sedated man undergoing EGD
  - HEENT: EGD in place
  - Chest: lungs clear with apnea
  - Cardiac: tachycadia
  - Abdomen: soft
  - Skin: cool
  - Neuro: sedated
- Nurse: calls team to room because of concern over patient condition

Critical actions
- Tell GI MD to stop procedure
- Manage airway
- Stop sedation

Transition point 1: 2 minutes

VS: unchanged with declining O_2 Sat

- Changes in physical exam: none
- GI MD resists stopping procedure, saying "Give me a few more minutes"
- Nurse: initially has his back, "he's the best in the business"
- Imaging: video playing of varices with hemorrhage

Critical actions
- Reinforce need to stop procedure
- Order IV fluid to treat hypotension

Transition point 2: 4 minutes

VS: unchanged

- Changes in physical exam/condition: none
- Labs: none available
- Imaging: none available
- Team must manage bloody airway, treat shock
- GI MD: at 4 minutes abandons procedure and leaves room

Critical actions
- Order blood transfusion given no response to IV fluid
- Manage airway

Transition point 3: 6 minutes

VS: BP 80/40, HR 130, HR 8, pulse oximetry 80%

- Changes in physical exam/patient condition
  - ▶ hemorrhage continues from oropharynx until treated
  - ▶ shock improves with initiation of massive transfusion protocol

Critical actions
- Insert Blakemore tube to control GI hemorrhage
- Order massive transfusion protocol

Transition point 4: final actions

VS: HR 130, HR intubated pulse oximetry 95%

- Changes in physical exam
  - ▶ appearance: unresponsive
  - ▶ if Blakemore tube placed, hemorrhage controlled
- Disposition: admit to ICU

Critical actions
- Reassess vital signs
- Admit to ICU

9. STIMULI

None.

10. BIBLIOGRAPHY

Chen ZJ, Freeman ML. Management of upper gastrointestinal bleeding emergencies: evidence-based medicine and practical considerations. *World J Emerg Med* 2011; 2:5–12.

Garcia-Tsao G, Bosch J. Management of varices and variceal hemorrhage in cirrhosis. *N Engl J Med* 2010; 362:823–32.

Transfer gone wrong: nasogastric tube in the trachea

Aaron Gingrich and Michael Falk

1. SCENARIO OVERVIEW

A patient arrives by EMS transfer from an outside hospital with acute respiratory distress syndrome (ARDS) because an NG tube was placed in the lungs. Patient was initially seen and evaluated in another hospital for GI bleeding. She presented to that ED with her EMS partner who was very unhappy with her care there. During the course of the evaluation at this ED, she has become increasing more ill and her EMS partner became more and more agitated with her care. Finally, he decides to "abscond" with his partner and they arrive in your ED for evaluation with her medical records.

On arrival in your ED, the EMS friend gives a history of her suffering from GI bleed and that when she first arrived at that "other ED" she was awake and alert and had no respiratory issues at all. Over the 3-hour course of her stay in that ED she suddenly developed difficulty breathing after he left her alone with "those quacks" to get some coffee and lunch. The team must manage the respiratory distress, identify the source of the problem and correct the errors.

2. TEACHING OBJECTIVES/DISCUSSION POINTS

Clinical and medical management

■ Critically re/evaluate all transfers
■ Review all records from other facility and confirm placement of indwelling catheters and IV tubes from another hospital: recognize improperly placed NG tube and IV lines
■ Recognize flash pulmonary edema as iatrogenic complication of NG lavage

Communication and teamwork

■ Obtain history from person accompanying patient and to review *all* available records/source of information
■ Appropriately redirect litigious family member and maintain professional demeanor
■ Discuss medical errors from another facility

3. SUPPLIES

NG tube, IV equipment, ETTs, laryngoscope with blades, IV supplies (normal saline bags and tubing) and fake medical record.

4. MOULAGE

NG tube placed in trachea, peripheral IV lines misplaced.

5. IMAGES AND LABS

XR23: NG tube in trachea

6. ACTORS (CONFEDERATES) AND THEIR ROLES

- Patient: as a voice.
- Nurse: removes and properly replaces new working IV lines only if directed to do so.
- Confederate: EMS friend.

7. CRITICAL ACTIONS

- Complete head-to-toe assessment
- Recognize need for new IV lines and pull old ones
- Obtain history from EMS friend
- Develop differential diagnosis for respiratory distress, diagnose iatrogenic flash pulmonary edema
- Intubate patient, start CPR, IV fluid, order blood products
- Recognize and discuss medical errors made by other hospital

8. TIMELINE

Time 0

VS: BP 100/50, HR 108, RR 24, O_2 Sat 93% RA, 38.0°C, EKG – sinus tachycardia

- Summary of initial presentation: middle-aged woman, groaning and responds to pain in non-purposeful fashion. She is pale, diaphoretic, breathing fast and hard, but is maintaining airway. NG tube in oropharynx
- Initial interventions: IV lines placed by other ED, prehospital 12-lead, etc.
- Physical exam
  - General: well nourished, well developed and pale female
  - HEENT: NG tube in trachea, jaw rigid and un-openable
  - Heart: sinus tachycardia
  - Chest: bilateral rales and tachypnea
  - Abdomen: non-distended
  - Extremities: no edema
  - Neuro: responds to painful stimuli with groans and purposeful movements

■ EMS friend: tells the team she is 48 years old, works as a paramedic. EMS friend is her crew partner. Patient has just been in the ED of County General Hospital for 3 hours and then absconded and was transferred by her partner because "They weren't taking care of her." Patient arrived at other facility with lower GI bleed and during the course of her evaluation she has become unresponsive and is not breathing well

Critical actions
• Complete physical examination

Transition point 1: 2 minutes

VS: BP 98/54, HR 110, RR 26, O_2 Sat 92% RA

■ Physical exam: patient has large bloody stool
■ Both peripheral IV lines are blown and any medication or fluids that are given do not work. If nurse asked to get new access and is unable, says "Why can't we just use the big ones already in place?"
■ EMS friend: reports that patient smokes heavily and drinks more coffee than anyone he knows. She has been complaining of abdomen pain for last month or so and has been eating antacids "like candy"

Critical actions
• Recognize need for new IV access and pull old ones
• Get history from friend
• Develop differential for respiratory distress

Transition point 2: 4 minutes

VS: BP 0/0, HR 0, RR 0, O_2 Sat 80% RA

■ Patient becomes hypotensive, and then goes pulseless; no BP
■ Initiate CPR and BMV on the patient
  ▶ establish IV access (can have team place IO access if desired)
  ▶ give epinephrine IV and normal saline bolus IV
■ If team tries to intubate without placing new IV lines they are unable to open the jaw
■ At this point the nurse is able to get new access after the first attempt to intubate; any newly placed IV lines work normally
■ EMS friend: fixated on complaining about care at the previous hospital, is agitated and asking for advice on how to sue. However, if directed, EMS partner reports she had initially come in with lots of dark blood in stool. Once they got her in to a room he stepped out for 30 minutes or so, to call her family, and he got back to find an NG tube in place and they were draining "like pink water out." That was when she got worse and had problems breathing. He has been fighting with them since then to get her here…"because that ER kills people!"

Critical actions
- Control or remove EMS friend, get additional history that he now gives
- Replace IV lines and pull NG if not done
- Intubate patient
- Start CPR; IV fluid; order blood products

Transition point 4: 6 minutes

VS: BP 0/0, HR 0, RR 0, O_2 Sat 80% RA – PEA

■ Continue CPR
  ▶ team should intubate patient using RSI protocol
  ▶ confirm placement of the ETT with at least two methods
  ▶ give second round of epinephrine and patient's VS should return at this point
■ Imaging: nurse finds X-ray from other facility and offers it to the team
■ Labs: Hgb/hemocrit: 8/24; labs otherwise normal
■ EMS friend: continues to be extremely upset, intrusive, collecting names of MD team members so they can "Help him sue that last hospital"

Critical actions
- Diagnose iatrogenic flash pulmonary edema
- Utilize PEEP on ventilator

Transition point 4: final actions

VS: BP 122/82, HR 120, RR 24, O_2 Sat 96% RA

■ Changes in physical exam: ROSC if ETT placed
■ EMS friend: returns if he has been removed. Is now well behaved and wants to discuss medical error made. Team *must* discuss the medical error that was made by the other hospital with EMS friend
■ Additional points: medical aspect of case should resolve and attention should be directed to a discussion with the EMS friend
■ Disposition: ICU

Critical actions
- Talk to EMS friend
- Disclose medical error made

9. STIMULI

XR23: NG tube in right lung (as part of "fake" medical record)

10. BIBLIOGRAPHY

Kalra J, Kalra N, Baniak N. Medical error, disclosure and patient safety: A global view of quality care. *Clin Biochem.* 2013; 46:1161–1169.
Silversides JA, Ferguson ND. Clinical review: acute respiratory distress syndrome – clinical ventilator management and adjunct therapy. *Crit Care* 2012; 17:225.

INFECTIOUS DISEASE

Septic shock secondary to pneumonia

Jacqueline A. Nemer and Julian Villar

1. SCENARIO OVERVIEW

A 74-year-old man with a history of asthma, type 1 diabetes, hypothyroidism and coronary artery disease was brought from home by ambulance for shortness of breath. According to his wife, the man had been less interactive and responsive over the past 3 days. He also had decreased appetite, less energy, moderate productive cough and appeared more short of breath. Prior to arrival O_2 saturation was 80% on RA, 88% on 4 L/min by NC. BP 88/56, HR 126, regular. Blood glucose is 110. The wife is in the room and is very upset, crying "Harry, Harry, don't go. You're everything!"

2. TEACHING OBJECTIVES/DISCUSSION POINTS

Clinical and medical management

- Understand differential diagnosis for shortness of breath and cough: infection, asthma, pulmonary embolus, metabolic disorder, MI, heart failure
- Understand the management of sepsis: definitions of systemic inflammatory response syndrome (SIRS) vs. sepsis vs. severe sepsis vs. septic shock
- Understand indications for ETT and its potential pitfalls

Communication and teamwork

- Team leader should maintain overall situational awareness and delegate specific tasks
- Professional interaction with nurses and consultants
- Appropriate management of nervous wife

3. SUPPLIES

Ultrasound, direct laryngoscope, ETT, syringe 10 mL (for tube)

4. MOULAGE

Mannequin dressed in pajamas; clothing and skin moist to mimic sweating.

5. IMAGES AND LABS

- EKG6: sinus tachycardia, no signs of ischemia or infarction
- XR10: CXR with multilobar pneumonia
- US3: poor volume status IVC
- US4: normal IVC after fluids, without respiratory variation
- CT chest: if ordered would show same, no pulmonary embolus

6. ACTORS (CONFEDERATES) AND THEIR ROLES

- Patient: mannequin which initially follows commands and is verbal, then becomes obtunded.
- Nurse: places patient on monitor, starts IV fluids, measures temperature, draws blood and gives medications.
- Consult: stalls, provides no help.
- Wife: initially provides some (useless) collateral information, then will become anxious and disruptive requiring redirection and soothing. If appropriate attention is given, wife will stop being disruptive.

7. CRITICAL ACTIONS

- Institute aggressive fluids
- Measure lactate
- Start broad-spectrum antibiotics
- Assess airway and intubation
- Use vasopressors for refractory hypotension

8. TIMELINE

Time 0

VS: BP 84/50, HR 128, RR 36, O_2 Sat 80% RA, 37.7°C (oral), EKG – sinus tachycardia

- Summary of initial presentation: 74-year-old man, history of asthma, productive cough and shortness of breath for a few days, now very short of breath and hypoxic in the field
- Initial interventions: nurse places patient on monitor, places one 18g IV line in left arm
- Physical exam
  - General: sweating, coughing, respiratory distress with single word answers
  - HEENT: dry lips, eyes open
  - Neck: no lymph nodes, no neck veins, rigid neck
  - Chest: diminished in all fields, coarse rhonchi, faint wheezes
  - Heart: tachycardic, regular rhythm, carotid and femoral pulses palpable, radials absent
  - Abdomen: soft, non-tender, non-distended
  - Neuro: non-focal, follows simple commands
  - Skin: sweaty, poor turgor

■ Wife: agitated, intrusive
■ Nurse: if asked, will place second IV line, draw blood for labs, start fluids, perform rectal temperature, convey patient's weight (100 kg, 220 lb), perform EKG (available at next time point), start antibiotics and vasopressors
■ Consultants: any and all are busy/unavailable/unhelpful

Critical actions
- Place on NRB
- Ask for rectal temperature (39.0°C)
- Ask for second IV line
- Redirect wife
- Give 20 mg/kg crystalloid
- Order lactate

Transition point 1: 2 minutes

VS: BP 84/50, HR 120–130, RR 38, O_2 Sat 77% RA

■ ▶ If placed on NRB: O_2 Sat 94%
   ▶ If placed on NC ≥4L/min: O_2 Sat 85%
   ▶ If placed on NC <4 L/min: arrest
   ▶ If not placed on O_2: arrest
■ Changes in physical exam: none
■ Labs: point of care blood sugar 92, Hgb 8.3
■ Imaging:
   ▶ EKG6: (if requested in previous time point)
   ▶ US3: poor volume status IVC
   ▶ CXR: not available yet if requested in previous or current time point
■ Wife: if team redirected and consoled in prior time point will no longer be an issue for rest of case; otherwise will continue to be intrusive and disruptive

Critical actions
- Consider and address differential
- Give nebulized albuterol for asthma

Transition point 2: 5 minutes

VS: BP see below, HR 120–130, RR 30, O_2 Sat 70% RA

■ ▶ if no second IV line and no fluids: arrest
   ▶ if no second IV line, fluids <20 mg/kg: BP 60/0
   ▶ if no second IV line, fluids ≥ 20 mg/kg: BP 70/30
   ▶ if second IV line placed and fluids appropriate: BP 88/56 (MAP 67)
   ▶ If albuterol given: O_2 Sat 90%
   ▶ If no nebs given: O_2 Sat fall 10%
■ Changes in physical exam/condition
   ▶ impending respiratory failure
   ▶ eyes closed, not following commands, non-verbal

■ Labs: lactate 5.2 mg/dL
■ Imaging: US3 (poor volume status IVC)

> **Critical actions**
> - Recognize septic shock (lactate >4, refractory hypotension)
> - Continue fluids, consider vasporessors
> - Recognize respiratory failure
> - Prepare to intubate

Transition point 3: 7 minutes

VS: systolic BP decreases by 10 mmHg, HR 120–130, RR 40, O_2 Sat 60% RA

■ Changes in physical exam/patient condition
  ▶ GCS 3
  ▶ if not preparing to intubate: arrest
  ▶ if no additional fluid bolus: arrest 30 seconds after paralytics given
  ▶ if additional fluid bolus and use versed/fentanyl or propofol: BP 50/0, may rescue with vasopressors otherwise patient arrests
  ▶ if additional fluid bolus, versed/fentanyl or propofol, but vasopressors being used: BP unchanged
  ▶ if additional fluid bolus and ketamine, no vasopressors: BP unchanged
  ▶ if additional fluid bolus, ketamine, vasopressors: BP 85/50 (MAP 61)
  ▶ if uses ketamine for induction but do not start vasopressors after intubation: BP 70/40 (MAP 50), which if left uncorrected leads to arrest
  ▶ if uses ketamine for induction and start vasopressors after intubation: BP 85/60
■ Labs:
  ▶ WBC 18 000, 20% bands
  ▶ Hbg 7.9
  ▶ hematocrit 23%
  ▶ creatinine 2.5
  ▶ other labs within normal limits, including cardiac biomarkers
■ Imaging: XR10 (CXR with multilobar pneumonia) if requested in first time point; US4, showing normal IVC after fluids

> **Critical actions**
> - Additional fluid bolus before intubation
> - Intubate
> - Start vasopressors
> - Critical action 3
> - Critical action 4

Transition point 4: final actions (if patient survives intubation)

VS: BP 85/60 (MAP 61), HR 100, mechanically ventilated

■ Changes in physical exam/condition:
  ▶ patient sedated and paralyzed
  ▶ if vasopressors increased: BP 100/70 (MAP 80)
■ Disposition: ICU

Critical actions
- Titrate vasopressors to MAP $\geq$65 mmHg
- Start antibiotics
- Consider blood transfusion
- Post-intubation CXR
- Admit to ICU
- Critical action 4

9. STIMULI

- EKG6: sinus tachycardia
- XR10: CXR with multilobar pneumonia
- US3: poor volume status IVC
- US4: normal IVC after fluids, without respiratory variation

10. BIBLIOGRAPHY

De Backer D et al. Dopamine versus norepinephrine in the treatment of septic shock: a meta-analysis. *Crit Care Med* 2012; 40:725–730.

Dellinger RP et al. Surviving Sepsis Campaign: international guidelines for management of severe sepsis and septic shock: 2012. *Crit Care Med* 2013; 41:580–637.

Rivers E et al. Early goal directed therapy in the treatment of severe sepsis and septic shock. *New Eng J Med* 2001; 345:1368–1377.

Rivers E et al. Early interventions in severe sepsis and septic shock: a review of the evidence one decade later. *Minerva Anestesiol* 2012; 78:712–724.

CASE 19

Altered mental status with hemorrhagic fever

Michael Falk

1. SCENARIO OVERVIEW

A 33-year-old man is brought in by EMS to a tertiary care center in the ED after being called by his significant other. The man was recently away in Africa working for an international aid organization and then visiting his partner's family in Panama. He has been complaining of high fevers, with a maximum temperature of 104.7°F at home, headache with eye pain, myalgias and joint pains. These symptoms started about 2 days after he returned home and have been getting worse. He has complained of worsening muscle and joint pains that are very severe and not relieved by NSAIDs that he was taking for the pain. His partner has not heard from him all day and after working late she came home to find him on the bathroom floor, minimally responsive. He arrives on 100% O_2 delivered by NRB mask and on a cardiac monitor.

During the case the partner is very upset *but* can be calmed by team member to provide history. Patient travels extensively, including his most recent trip to Africa, from which he returned 2 weeks ago. He has had a number of tropical diseases before because of his work, and all she remembers is malaria and when prompted dengue.

2. TEACHING OBJECTIVES/DISCUSSION POINTS

Clinical and medical management

- Identify a differential diagnosis of fever and AMS in patient with high risk (travel)
- Identify the need for and take universal precautions
- Develop differential diagnosis for hemorrhagic fever
- Recognize and begin resuscitation for patient in shock
- Recognize and perform RSI for airway stabilization

Communication and teamwork

- Team leader establishes clear roles (which includes assigning a person to talk with the partner and get travel and PMH)
- Team identifies the need for and establishes universal precautions

■ Team identifies and alerts the appropriate people to deal with infectious hemorrhagic fever
■ Lastly, team should identify and establish a "safe" area for this patient that decreases risk of spread to others in the ER

3. SUPPLIES

Pajamas, IV supplies.

4. MOULAGE

Patient should have dried vomit/blood around mouth and face. He should have number of bruises on various parts of his body that are relatively "fresh" and petechiae. Needs to "leak blood" around IV access site at some point during the case to make the hemorrhagic fever obvious. To do this, place an IV line and use moulage blood around the IV catheter and the skin. Cover it with some kind of opaque dressing and have the nurse remove it during the case when you want to identify the issue.

5. IMAGES AND LABS

■ No images are necessary but consider XR1 (normal male CXR)
■ Labs: CBC, BMP, LFTs, ABG, clotting

6. ACTORS (CONFEDERATES) AND THEIR ROLES

■ Patient: mannequin.
■ Nurse: should be knowledgeable and very helpful.
■ Consult: infectious disease specialist should be called; if called immediately identifies the need for strict isolation and hemorrhagic fever precautions. If GI or other service consulted, can have them suggest infectious disease consult.
■ Partner: should be very upset; they were just engaged while visiting parents in Panama and is now distraught. The partner *can* be calmed *if* a team member is provided to help talk to her and if she is calmed she will then give the travel history and the fact that he has had dengue before (making shock and hemorrhagic fever more likely) and can mention that his/her parents mentioned there was a "outbreak" of some kind where they were in Panama.

7. CRITICAL ACTIONS

1. Identify and treat patient in shock
2. Recognize infectious hemorrhagic fever and establish appropriate precautions for the team
3. Identify the appropriate authorities for a case of infectious hemorrhagic fever
4. Ensure rest of the ED is safe and that patient is "isolated"
5. Establish and maintain definitive airway because of patient's deteriorating condition

8. TIMELINE

Time 0

VS: BP 70/42, HR 124, RR 100% NRB, 39.7°C, EKG – sinus tachycardia

■ Summary of initial presentation: patient brought in by EMS with partner for "vomiting blood." He is groaning and responds slowly to painful stimuli. He has cap refill times of >4 seconds and mottled appearance with bruises
■ Initial interventions: an IV line placed by EMS (can have this one "prepped" for leaking blood) and started on IV fluids
■ Physical exam
  ▶ General: pronounced facial flushing, has shirt and pants on with bloody emesis on front of shirt, and responds to questions by groaning and minimal non-specific movements to pain
  ▶ HEENT: as above and slight bleeding from gums if they check his mouth or if they decide to place NG tube (nurse can comment on)
  ▶ Chest: lungs are CTA, tachycardic
  ▶ Abdomen: soft, non-tender, non-distended and hypoactive bowel sounds
  ▶ Skin: extensive petechiae on extremities and purpura with delayed cap refill and mottled appearance
  ▶ Extremities: normal except above
  ▶ Neuro: groaning non-specifically to stimuli and responds minimally to pain
■ Nurse: very helpful and should mention bruising and petechiae if team does not identify these findings
■ Partner: hysterical but can be controlled

Critical actions
- Place on monitor
- Establish second IV line and send labs
- Initiate fluid bolus
- Control fever

Transition point 1: 2 minutes

VS: BP 78/46, HR 118, RR 100% on NRB with 100% O_2

■ No exam changes
■ Should consider second bolus of IV fluid
■ If NG tube placed, patient should develop bleeding around NG site and fresh blood drawn back from tube
■ Imaging: if CXR requested, provide XR1 (normal male CXR)
■ Nurse: has established second IV line and labs are off. If not identified by team, the nurse should again mention the bruising etc. and then show them the EMS IV site
■ Partner: calmer and starts to give travel history and that he has been sick since he returned

Critical actions
- Establish travel history
- Consider second bolus
- Begin to recognize that patient has "bleeding" problem

Transition point 2: 4 minutes

VS: BP 78/48, HR 118, RR 22 on 100% NRB

- ■ Changes in physical exam/condition: patient is becoming more unresponsive and now does *not* respond to pain
- ■ Consider/give third bolus of fluids
- ■ Team should identify need for possible airway intervention
- ■ Team should now be considering "uncommon" cause of bleeding and fever (for the developed world at least) and should establish universal precautions, mask, gown, gloves, etc., if not done
- ■ Request packed RBCs, platelets and plasma from blood bank
- ■ Consult infectious disease unit
- ■ Labs: see below
- ■ Nurse: should be pushing team to activate appropriate resources for such a high-risk case, "I really think I need to call my nurse manager and infection control"
- ■ Partner: much calmer and should have provided full history by now, including PMH and the "outbreak" near where parents live

Critical actions
- Establish universal precautions
- Consider third bolus
- Preparation for RSI

Transition point 3: 6 minutes

VS: BP 86/52, HR 110, RR 22, O_2 Sat 92% on NRB, gurgling

- ■ Changes in physical exam/patient condition: completely non-responsive and not maintaining airway
- ■ RSI with appropriate medications given hypotension and worries about sepsis
- ■ Confirm placement using *at* least two techniques, one *must* be $ETCO_2$ detector
- ■ Infectious diseases consult should call back: if team has not made the call, should advise team of infection risk and the need to activate appropriate protocols
- ■ Imaging: XR3, CXR confirming intubation if requested
- ■ Partner: wants to be kept in the loop and team should tell him/her what is happening

Critical actions
- Perform RSI with correct medication
- Activate protocols for high infection risk

Transition point 4: final actions

VS: BP 86/53, HR 110, RR vented, O_2 Sat 100% RA

- Changes in physical exam: patient is intubated
- Should consider transfusion at this time
- Call and sign out to ICU and *must* identify need for negative pressure room
- Partner: team leader should have conversation with partner about patient's condition and what to expect
- MICU: accepts patient

Critical actions
- Sign out to MICU
- Consider blood transfusion
- Discussion with partner

10. STIMULI

- Consider XR1 (normal male CXR) and/or XR3 (normal male intubated CXR)
- Labs

Parameter	Value	Comment
CBC		
WBC	1.7	
Hgb/hematocrit	11.3/34	Hemoconcentration from plasma leak, which is seen in shock associated with Dengue fever
Platlets	37	Leukopenia is associated with dengue; platelets consistent with hemorrhagic fever
BMP		
Sodium	127	Dengue lowers sodium concentrations
BUN/creatinine	36/1.2	Plasma leak and distributive shock
Albumin	2.1	Plasma leak and distributive shock
LFTs		
AST	546	
ALT	477	
ABG	Metabolic acidosis	
PT/PTT	18/41	

11. BIBLIOGRAPHY

Centers for Disease Control and Prevention. *Viral Hemorrhagic Fevers*. Atlanta, GA: National Center for Infectious Diseases, Centers for Disease Control and Prevention, 2013 (http://www.cdc.gov/ncidod/dvrd/spb/mnpages/dispages/vhf.htm, accessed 31 July 2014).

Gubler DJ. Dengue and dengue hemorrhagic fever. *Clin Microbiol Rev* 1998; 11:480–496.

Rothman AL, Sriakiathachorn A, Kalayanarooj S. Clinical manifestations and diagnosis of dengue virus infections. *UpToDate* 2013 (http://www.uptodate.com/contents/clinical-presentation-and-diagnosis-of-dengue-virus-infections?source=search_result&search=dengue±fever&selectedTitle=1%7E42, accessed 31 July 2014).

Tetany in a home body piercer

Christopher Sampson and Jason Wagner

1. SCENARIO OVERVIEW

A 35-year-old man with schizophrenia presents via EMS with body shaking. Onset of whole body shaking, worse with bright light and noise. Wallet with psychiatry appointment card reveals name and scheduled haloperidol injections.

2. TEACHING OBJECTIVES/DISCUSSION POINTS

Clinical and medical management

- Understand differential for limb shaking
- Know appropriate treatment for tetany

Communication and teamwork

- Team leader named at start of case
- Team leader assigns roles

3. SUPPLIES

Nipple ring with moulage, appointment card in wallet for scheduled haloperidol decanoate injection, intraosseus needle driver.

4. MOULAGE

Nipple ring on mannequin with surrounding cellulitis.

5. IMAGES AND LABS

- EKG1: sinus tachycardia
- Labs: CBC, BMP

6. ACTORS (CONFEDERATES) AND THEIR ROLES

■ EMS: provides HPI at patient arrival.
■ Girlfriend: provides additional HPI if needed.

7. CRITICAL ACTIONS

■ Airway support
■ Placement of IO given inability to place IV line because of the patient shaking
■ Administer tetanus immunoglobulin
■ Administer antibiotics
■ Admit to ICU

8. TIMELINE

Time 0

VS: BP 170/90, HR 135, RR 22, O_2 Sat 100% RA, 38.0°C, EKG – sinus tachycardia

■ Summary of initial presentation: patient brought in by EMS on stretcher; patient is agitated and screaming and yells at staff to turn off lights and not make so much noise
■ Initial interventions: EMS unable to obtain IV access
■ Physical exam
  ▶ General: agitated man, shaking every few seconds, in jeans and T-shirt
  ▶ HEENT: grinning mouth
  ▶ Neck: stiffness, resists movement
  ▶ Chest: left nipple ring with surrounding erythema and pustular drainage; CTA bilaterally
  ▶ Abdomen: tense
  ▶ Skin: warm, diaphoresis
  ▶ Neuro: frequent contractions of muscles
■ EMS: provides patient report

Critical actions
• Assess patient

Transition point 1: 2 minutes

VS: BP 165/92, HR 130, RR 20, O_2 Sat 98% RA

■ Patient begins shaking again and screams, yelling about the lights in the room
■ Unable to obtain IV access because shaking so much
■ Nurse is concerned about her own safety given the patient's movements

Critical actions
• IO access placed
• Consider restraints for safety of staff/patient
• Completely disrobe patient

Transition point 2: 3 minutes

VS: BP 174/96, HR 140, RR 24, O_2 Sat 99% RA

■ Patient begins shaking again, which will resolve briefly with benzodiazepine administration
■ Nurse locates wallet with haloperidol card in pocket
■ Team may consider benztropine, diphenhydramine, more benzodiazepine

Critical actions
• Order benzodiazepines
• Considers tardive dyskinesia in the differential

Transition point 3: 4 minutes

VS: BP 172/94, HR 138, RR 22 98% RA

■ Patient develops laryngospasm and become hypoxic
■ O_2 Sat drop to 82%
■ If not intubated will go into respiratory arrest
   ▶ patient needs to be preoxygenated
   ▶ Sim operator should lock jaw and allow time to progress as it would if patient received paralytic chosen by team
■ Girlfriend: arrives and provides history of home body piercing that became infected

Critical actions
• Airway management
• RSI with laryngospasm

Transition point 4: final actions

VS: BP 136/94, HR 110, RR 14, O_2 Sat 100% RA

■ Patient intubated, paralyzed
■ Additional points
   ▶ administer tetanus immunoglobulin, antibiotics
   ▶ discuss expected course with girlfriend
■ Disposition: ICU admission; accepted to ICU only if correct diagnosis is made

Critical actions
• ICU admission
• Tetanus immunoglobulin administered

9. STIMULI

- EKG1: sinus tachycardia
- Labs:
  - ▶ elevated WBC, 13
  - ▶ normal electrolytes

10. BIBLIOGRAPHY

Richardson JP, Knight AL. The management and prevention of tetanus. *J Emerg Med* 1993; 11:737–42.

Sampson CS. Tetanus after home piercing. *J Emerg Med* 2013; 45:95–6.

Pediatric myocarditis

Andrew Schmidt and Lisa Jacobson

1. SCENARIO OVERVIEW

A 5-year-old boy presents with non-English-speaking parents who are concerned because he is fatigued. Evaluation reveals evidence of acute heart failure secondary to myocarditis. Attempts to transfer patient to referral center are met with resistance due to uninsured and undocumented status of patient.

2. TEACHING OBJECTIVES/DISCUSSION POINTS

Clinical and medical management

■ Recognition of cardiogenic shock in a pediatric patient
■ Initial resuscitation of pediatric acute heart failure
■ Management of fulminant myocarditis
■ Recognition of need for specialized/intensive care

Communication and teamwork

■ Utilization of translational services
■ Efficient communication with consulting services

3. SUPPLIES

Pediatric mannequin, pediatric airway supplies, translator phone, consent form.

4. MOULAGE

None.

5. IMAGES AND LABS

■ EKG8: pediatric tachycardia
■ XR11: pediatric CXR

■ Labs as given below
■ Consent form

6. ACTORS (CONFEDERATES) AND THEIR ROLES

■ Nurse: nervous about caring for a child, pushes the issue of consent if not addressed by team.
■ Parents: non-English speaking, visibly concerned.
■ Child: as a voice.
■ Interpreter/translation: phone line.
■ Consulting transfer team (phone): refers team to "transfer center" at his/her institution.
■ Transfer line at referral center: concerned about cost, insurance, citizenship.

7. CRITICAL ACTIONS

■ Recognize a critically ill child
■ Recognize hypotension in a child and administer appropriate initial bolus of IV fluids
■ Place child on monitor and administer O_2
■ Utilize translation line to communicate further with parents and gain any necessary consent
■ Recognize unstable arrhythmia
■ Treat unstable arrhythmia with proper cardioversion
■ Contact hospital with ICU

8. TIMELINE

Time 0

VS: BP 90/45, HR 165, RR 35, O_2 Sat 93% on 2 L NC, 101°F, EKG – sinus tachycardia

■ Summary of initial presentation: 5-year-old boy arrives by private car with parents, who do not speak English. Child speaks English but appears very fatigued and is slow to respond. He complains of loss of energy, decreased appetite and chest pain. He denies taking any medications at home and denies any ingestions
■ Physical exam
  ▶ General: oriented x3, lethargic
  ▶ HEENT: normal
  ▶ Neck: JVD
  ▶ Heart: diminished pulses, aortic regurgitation murmur, muffled heart sounds, tachycardic, displaced point of maximal impulse
  ▶ Chest: tachypneic, rales
  ▶ Extremities: cool
  ▶ Skin: clammy and pale
■ Parents: only statements they can make in English are "He's tired," "He's feverish" and "He's never been sick before"

Tranisition 1: 3 minutes

VS: BP 80/35, HR 165, RR 40, O_2 Sat 88% on any O_2, 101°F

- Changes in physical exam/condition: Overall decompensation despite fluid boluses or pressors
- Labs: CBC, BMP, cardiac markers, lactate, ESR (see Supplies)
- Imaging: none available
- Nurse: if team attempts to do any invasive procedures (central line, intubation), nurse will press for consent from parents

Transition 2: 4 minutes

VS: BP 75/30, HR 165, RR 40 O_2 Sat 86% on any O_2, 101°F

- Changes in physical exam/condition: minimal improvements will result from intubation, central line access, pressors, or diuresis
- Imaging:
  ▶ XR11: pediatric CXR
  ▶ EKG8: pediatric sinus tachycardia
  ▶ Verbalize: echo gives left ventricular dilation, global hypokinesis, no effusion

  Nurse: if team attempts to do any invasive procedures (central line, intubation), nurse will press for consent from parents

Transition 3: 5 minutes

VS: BP 70/30, HR 200, EKG – ventricular tachycardia

- ▶ if intubated: RR 40, O_2 Sat 88%
  ▶ if intubated: RR 60, O_2 Sat 80%
- Changes in physical exam/condition: EKG ventricular tachycardia (with pulses) converts to sinus tachycardia with cardioversion

Time 4: final actions

■ If team has not done so, at this point nurse prompts call for transfer since hospital does not have a PICU

■ Upon calling for consulting service, advised that they only accept transfers through their referral service. If team calls consulting service again directly they will continue to refuse and hang up

■ If team calls referral line, they will be asked for insurance or citizenship documentation. If team states there is none, referral center refuses transfer

VS: same as previous

Changes in physical exam/condition:

■ ▶ patient continues to decompensate despite IV fluid or pressors
  ▶ hypoxia refractory to intubation with FiO$_2$ 100%
■ Parents: if asked about insurance or citizenship documentation, state they have none (all communications must be done through translation line)

> **Critical actions**
> • Contact hospital with PICU
> • Continue aggressive resuscitation

9. STIMULI

■ EKG8: pediatric tachycardia
■ XR11: pediatric CXR
■ Consent form
■ Labs
  ▶ CBC: WBC 15 with lymph 80%; otherwise normal
  ▶ BMP: sodium 125, otherwise normal
  ▶ cardiac markers: troponin: 0.08, creatine kinase normal, creatine kinase-MB normal
  ▶ lactate: 3 mol/L
  ▶ ESR: 50

10. BIBLIOGRAPHY

Freedman SB, Haladyn JK, Floh A et al. Pediatric myocarditis: emergency department clinical findings and diagnostic evaluation. *Pediatrics* 2007; 120:1278–1285.

Levine MC, Klugman D, Teach SJ. Update on myocarditis in children. *Curr Opin Pediatr* 2010; 22: 278–283.

Scott MM, Macias CG, Jefferies JL, Kim JJ, Price JF. Acute heart failure syndromes in the pediatric emergency department. *Pediatrics* 2009; 124:e898–e904.

Yee LL, Meckler GD. Pediatric heart disease: acquired heart disease. In Tintinalli JE, Stapczynski JS, Cline DM et al. eds. *Tintinalli's Emergency Medicine: A Comprehensive Study Guide*, 7th edn. New York: McGraw-Hill, 2011, Ch. 122B.

Neonatal herpes simplex viral meningo/encephalitis

Kelvin Harold and Lisa Jacobson

1. SCENARIO OVERVIEW

An 11-day-old infant boy brought to the ED by his mother for 1 day history of the non-specific complaints of poor feeding, "not looking quite right" and breathing funny. Mother denies fever, vomiting, diarrhea, cough, or rash at triage. The patient is severely septic, in significant respiratory distress and progresses through septic shock, presumably from encephalitis/meningitis. Although there is no specific etiological diagnosis made through the simulation there are several key decisions that should be initiated.

2. TEACHING OBJECTIVES/DISCUSSION POINTS

Clinical and medical management

- Recognition of respiratory distress in the neonate
- Management of respiratory distress in the neonate
- Recognition of the septic neonate
- Management of the septic neonate
- Airway management in the neonate
- Recognize that maternal history for herpes simplex virus (HSV) is negative the majority of the time
- Indications for acyclovir in the ill/septic neonate

3. SUPPLIES

No case-specific supplies.

4. MOULAGE

None.

5. IMAGES AND LABS

EKG9: neonatal sinus tachycardia, 180s
XR12: normal neonatal CXR

6. ACTORS (CONFEDERATES) AND THEIR ROLES

■ Patient: hi-fidelity neonatal/infant mannequin.
■ Nurse: assists in medication dosing, supply gathering, basic implementation.
■ Consult: NICU/PICU: will accept but please continue to stabilize patient before transfer.
■ Mother ± father: confused, minimally helpful, unconcerned.

7. CRITICAL ACTIONS

Objective 1: recognize neonatal respiratory distress
Objective 2: resuscitate a decompensated neonate with appropriate access and fluids
Objective 3: manage parental expectations with compassion
Objective 4: recognize need to treat, and appropriately treat for sepsis and meningitis/encephalitis
Objective 5: consider hypoglycemia, in addition to infection as source of shock in neonate
Objective 6: choose correct medications and equipment for neonatal intubation

8. TIMELINE

Time 0

VS: BP 51/27, HR 180, RR 80, O_2 Sat 92% RA, 94.5°F (34.7°C), EKG – heart rate in 180s

■ Summary of initial presentation: toxic appearing neonate, lying on bed with grunting respirations; heart rate in 180s, saturation the low 90s on room air
■ Initial interventions: none, arrived in mother's arms
■ Physical exam
  ▶ HEENT: flat fontanelle, PERRL, clear tympanic membranes, oropharynx without lesions
  ▶ Neck: supple without lymphadenopathy
  ▶ Chest: intercostal retractions, lungs clear to auscultation
  ▶ Heart: tachycardic, no audible murmur, capillary refill prolonged at 3 seconds
  ▶ Abdomen: distended, liver edge palpable to 3 cm below the right costal margin
  ▶ Genitourinary/rectal: uncircumcised, no lesions, normal tone if performed, guaiac negative
  ▶ Skin: mottled, no lesions
  ▶ Neuro: lethargic, responds to stimuli with feeble cry and moves all extremities equally

Critical action
• Recognize respiratory distress and provide supplemental O_2

Transition point 1: 2 minutes

VS: BP 51/27, HR 180, RR 92% RA

■ Airway: patent currently
■ Breathing: initiate supplemental O_2 with 100% NRB
  ▶ if not instituted, O_2 saturation will dip into the high 80s

▶ if O_2 saturation fall not addressed within 2–3 minutes, patient will develop bradycardia

▶ if O_2 is provided with 100% NRB, O_2 Sat will improve to high 90s (97–99%)

■ Circulation: establish IO access (will have difficult IV access and require placement of IO) and initiate rapid infusion of normal saline 10 mL/kg

■ Additional actions: bedside blood glucose should be checked; if checked, it is equal to 181 mg/dL

Critical actions
- Establish IV/IO access
- Provide rapid infusion of normal saline
- Check bedside serum glucose

Transition point 2: 3 minutes

VS (if above interventions are initiated the vitals will improve): BP 59/31, HR 180, RR 72, O_2 Sat 98% on 15 L/min, 94.5°F (34.7°C)

■ Orders:

▶ blood for laboratory studies, including CBC, electrolytes, BUN, creatinine, glucose, LFTs, ABG/VBG, coagulation profile (PT, PTT, INR), blood culture; consider lactate

▶ Urinalysis and culture

▶ Portable CXR

■ Patient has brief apneic episode: small drop in O_2 saturation; apnea resolves with stimulation

■ If LP is attempted at this point, the patient will desaturate and become apneic as is not yet stable enough for this intervention

■ Initiate IV (IO) antibiotics: ampicillin 100 mg/kg and cefotaxime 50 mg/kg

■ Labs: urinalysis is negative for leukocytes, nitrite, protein, blood; specific gravity 1.030

Critical actions
- Appropriate antibiotics
- Order CXR
- Recognize apnea

Transition point 4: 4 minutes

VS: BP 59/31, HR 180, RR: 72, O_2 Sat 92% on 15 L/min, 94.5°F (34.7°C)

■ Additional prenatal and birth history provided by mother: 19-year-old G1P1, one prenatal visit with uncomplicated spontaneous vaginal delivery, full-term infant now with 1 day history of poor feeding, pale appearance, breathing hard; mother denies any knowledge of infections during pregnancy

■ Decompensation: as mother is providing history, patient will develop apnea and O_2 Sat will start to decrease, not initially responsive to stimulation; at this point mother will panic

■ Airway management: initiate BVM ventilation. Patient will respond and start spontaneous respiration again, but the decision to intubate the patient should be made now
  ▶ drug choices for RSI: induction agent etomidate or ketamine; paralytic succinylcholine or rocuronium
  ▶ equipment choice: need to know the appropriate sized ETT or have a system to determine the appropriate size (e.g. Broselow–Luten tape)
  ▶ Team should set ventilator and decide what to use for sedation/comfort

---

Critical actions
- Decision to intubate
- Stimulate for apnea
- RSI with appropriate equipment and drugs

Transition point 5: 6 minutes

VS: BP none, HR 180, RR 72, O_2 Sat 97% on 100% FiO_2, 94.5°F (34.7°C)

■ Post-intubation pulse very weak: only central pulse palpable
■ Repeat BP at this point is not detectable
■ Need to institute second bolus normal saline (10 mL/kg): give it IV push
■ Some response to fluid bolus; BP improves to 40s/20s
■ May repeat fluid bolus, but BP is resistant to fluids
  ▶ need to start inotrope at this point (dopamine vs. other agent)
  ▶ BP improves with appropriate inotrope
■ Mother: if not incorporated into process becomes very nervous, tearful, difficult to manage

---

Critical actions
- Recognize and manage hypotension

Transition point: final actions

VS: BP 73/42, HR 180, RR 72 O_2, 94.5°F (34.7°C)

■ Should consider LP at this time
■ CXR: nothing abnormal detected
■ Lab results
  ▶ CBC: WBC 24, Hgb 10.1, hematocrit 29%, platelets 127
  ▶ BMP: sodium 130, potassium 5.4, chloride 99, bicarbonate 6, BUN 22, creatinine 0.8, glucose 194
  ▶ PT, PTT, INR: all within normal limits
  ▶ LFTs: AST 2464, ALP 379, bilirubin 3.5 mg/dL
  ▶ ABG: pH 7.1, PCO_2 22, PO_2 271, O_2 Sat 99%
  ▶ Lactate: 5.3 mmol/L
■ Combination of hypothermia, septic appearance, respiratory distress and abnormal LFTs should prompt suspicion for disseminated HSV at this point. It is acceptable

if LP is deferred due to concerns for patient's stability. If LP is deferred, acyclovir should be started (20 mg/kg IV)

■ If LP is performed, the results are as follows: WBC 108 (20% polymorphonuclear leukocytes, 80% mononuclear leukocytes), RBC 47, glucose 57, protein 115

■ LP results should prompt initiation of acyclovir if not already initiated

■ PICU consultant can push diagnosis if by final actions the team has not recognized it

Critical actions
- Confirm patient has received/is receiving all antimicrobials
- Review most current vital signs
- PICU admission

9. STIMULI

XR12: normal neonatal CXR, wet read

EKG9: neonatal sinus tachycardia

10. BIBLIOGRAPHY

Caviness AC *et al.* Cost-effectiveness analysis of herpes simplex virus testing and treatment strategies in febrile neonates. *Archives of Pediatrics and Adolescent Medicine* 2008; 162:665–74.

Dellinger RP *et al.* Surviving Sepsis Campaign: International Guidelines for Management of Severe Sepsis and Septic Shock: 2008. *Critical Care Medicine* 2008; 36:296–327.

El-wiher N *et al.* Management and treatment guidelines for sepsis in pediatric patients. *Open Inflammation Journal* 2011; 7:101–9.

Jones CA *et al.* Antiviral agents for treatment of herpes simplex virus infection in neonates. *Cochrane Database of Systematic Reviews* 2013; (8)CD004206.

SECTION 5

NEUROCRITICAL CARE

Traumatic brain injury

Nikita K. Joshi and Yasuharu Okuda

1. SCENARIO OVERVIEW

A 75-year-old man, PMH hypertension and dementia, was walking his dog with his niece, tripped on a hole in the street while crossing and hit the side of his head on the curb. He had loss of consciousness at the time but recovered and went home, then started to become confused. EMS called 1 hour after the event; man brought in by ambulance on backboard and collar. He is confused and agitated, trying to take off his collar and get off the stretcher, calling for his dog Spotty. Allows IV access but must be sedated for rest of exam and management. After sedation, becomes increasingly agitated and ultimately unresponsive with posturing. He needs advanced airway but is a difficult airway. Head CT shows large epidural hematoma with midline shift.

2. TEACHING OBJECTIVES/DISCUSSION POINTS

Clinical and medical management

- Performing primary and secondary survey in patient with traumatic brain injury
- Treatment of acutely agitated patient with traumatic brain injury
- Airway management in head trauma
- Avoid hypoxia, BVM technique
- ICP monitoring
- Management of ICP and BP

Communication and teamwork

- Performing thorough history and physical exam with an agitated and altered patient
- Communicating with difficult consultants

3. SUPPLIES

- IV fluid
- Syringes for medication administration
- Cervical collar

- Gauze
- Spinal neutralization board
- Non-invasive airway supplies: nasal trumpet, NRB
- Intubation supplies: BVM, ETT, stylet, blade and handle, suction, back-up airway

4. MOULAGE

Abrasions and blood on the extremities and forehead; 4 cm hematoma over the left temporal region of the head.

5. IMAGES AND LABS

- CT5: epidural hematoma with midline shift
- Labs: CBC, BMP, clotting, type and screen

6. ACTORS (CONFEDERATES) AND THEIR ROLES

- Patient: mannequin who is agitated, combative, refusing to cooperate with exam.
- Niece: very worried about her uncle, anxious that she should have called for EMS immediately.
- EMS: gives brief history of finding the patient in the home, and the difficulty of putting the patient on the board and in the collar.
- Nurse: helpful and cooperative with the team.

7. CRITICAL ACTIONS

- Obtaining rapid fingerstick blood
- Prepare for difficult airway management
- Safely manage a difficult and altered patient
- Avoid and manage hypotension
- Adhere to ATLS protocol
- Obtaining stat head CT

8. TIMELINE

Time 0–4 minutes

VS: BP 100/74, HR 20, RR 120, O_2 Sat 94% on O_2, 36.4°C (tympanic), fingerstick glucose 85 (must ask), EKG – sinus tachycardia

- Summary of initial presentation: 75-year-old man PMH hypertension, dementia tripped on a hole in the street and hit the side of his head on the curb. He had LOC at the time but recovered and went home, with some assistance by his niece, then started to become confused. EMS called by niece 1 hour post-event; man brought in by ambulance on backboard and collar. He is now in ED confused and agitated, trying to take off his collar and get off the stretcher, calling for his dog Spotty. Team is encouraged to sedate the patient by the nurse
- Physical exam

- ▶ General: agitated and anxious, oriented x1, trying to get out of stretcher to look for his dog, pulling at his cervical collar; refuses to allow intubation if the team tries to intubate him immediately
- ▶ HEENT: large 4 cm hematoma over his left temporal area, pupils 2 mm equal/ reactive
- ▶ Neck: in collar, no obvious signs of injury
- ▶ Chest: CTA
- ▶ Heart: regular
- ▶ Abdomen: normal
- ▶ Skin: abrasions on knees and left hand
- ▶ Neuro: grossly non-focal; not following all commands
- ■ Initial interventions:
  - ▶ IV line placed in AC 20G without difficulty
  - ▶ blood sent off for tests: CBC, CMP, PT/PTT, type and screen
  - ▶ head CT ordered
- ■ EMS: describes the difficulty of getting the patient to comply with their exam, of placing the cervical collar and remaining on the back board; quickly exits
- ■ Niece: gives full detailed history of patient's traumatic event, wishes that she could have brought the dog to the ED; she feels that if she brought the dog then the patient might be more willing to comply. Tries to get her uncle to comply with the exam, but does not want the medical team to hurt the patient; does not allow team to intubate him right away if the team tries to because she says her uncle is still talking
- ■ Nurse: helpful and assisting with all orders; recommends sedation such as halo-peridol/ lorazepam to assist with exam

---

Critical actions
- Obtain detailed history regarding traumatic head injury
- Perform thorough neurological examination
- Perform ATLS compliant trauma examination including primary and secondary survey with log roll and rectal examination
- Treatment of agitation in a patient with traumatic brain injury

---

Transition point 2: 4 minutes

VS: BP 140/84, HR 10, RR 60 (Cheyne–Stokes), O_2 Sat 91% on O_2

- ■ Physical exam: after given sedation, patient becomes increasingly confused and unresponsive, starts to posture: decerebrate positioning
- ■ Team must obtain definitive airway based on patient's change in mental status:
  - ▶ consider RSI and LOAD
  - ▶ if given full dose etomidate: then BP decreases
  - ▶ if given full dose propofol: then BP decreases
  - ▶ if given ketamine: then BP increases
  - ▶ must assemble airway adjuncts
  - ▶ must demonstrate good BVM bagging technique
  - ▶ intubation 1 fails if no airway adjunct

▶ intubation 2 fails if no airway adjunct

▶ intubation 3 success

■ CT calls for patient:

▶ if he is not intubated, CT technician states that he cannot go over to scanner because he sounds "unstable" over the phone

▶ if he is intubated: CT technician states that he can go to scanner

■ If he is intubated: BP will drop to 90/54, only responds to 1 L IV bolus of normal saline

■ Niece: very frightened by patient's appearance after sedation, wants to understand what is happening

■ Nurse: helpful and compliant with all orders given by team

Critical actions
- Recognize decompensation state in patient
- Recognize difficult airway by assembling airway adjuncts
- Obtain definitive airway
- Maintain cervical spine immobilization for intubation of trauma patient
- Treat hypotension as a result of intubation and oversedation

Transition point 3: 6 minutes

VS: BP dependent upon sedation and RSI drugs, HR 60, RR 10 intubated 100% on ventilator

■ Physical exam: sedated and paralyzed, otherwise unchanged

■ CT calls: tells the team that there is something wrong with the head CT; images show a large left-sided epidural hematoma

■ Team needs to change ventilator settings for hyperventilation, discuss use of mannitol, discuss use of hypertonic saline, raising head of the bed to 30 degrees

■ If neurosurgery is consulted: they call to the ED and request summary of patent's history and ED management; agree with disposing to the neurosurgery ICU

■ Niece: demands to know what an epidural hematoma is

■ Nurse: helpful, assisting in performing orders

Critical actions
- Treatment of intracranial hemorrhage
- Must obtain neurosurgery consult
- Must disposition the patient to the neurosurgery ICU

9. STIMULI

■ CT5: epidural hematoma with midline shift

■ Labs

▶ CBC: WBC 13, Hgb 9, hematocrit 30, platelets 200

▶ BMP: sodium 133. potassium 4.2, chloride 108, bicarbonate 23, BUN 15, creatinine 2.3, glucose 140, calcium 9.0

▶ clotting: PT/PTT 12/33

▶ type and screen

10. BIBLIOGRAPHY

Chan EW, Taylor DM, Phillips GA, Castle DJ, Kong DC. Intravenous droperidol or olanzapine as an adjunct to midazolam for the acutely agitated patient: a multicenter, randomized, double-blind, placebo-controlled clinical trial. *Ann Emerg Med* 2013; 1:72–81.

Chesnut RM, Temkin N, Carney N et al. A trail of intracranial-pressure monitoring in traumatic brain injury. *N Engl J Med* 2012; 367:2471–2481.

Wakai I, Roberts G, Schierhout G, et al. Mannitol for acute traumatic brain injury. *Cochrane Database Syst Rev* 2007; (1): CD001049.

Status epilepticus

Nikita K. Joshi and Yasuharu Okuda

1. SCENARIO OVERVIEW

A 31-year-old obese woman is brought in by the EMS for generalized tonic–clonic seizures to the ED. EMS were called to a coffee shop where witnesses said patient was seen reading a book, fell to her right side on the chair and started to shake all over and foam at the mouth. She was placed on NRB by BLS and transferred to ED. En route, she had second seizure lasting 1 minute without return to baseline. Time from onset of first seizure to arrival in the ED is 10 minutes. Patient will continue to seize in the ED, requiring the team to recognize and manage status epilepticus.

2. TEACHING OBJECTIVES/DISCUSSION POINTS

Clinical and medical management

■ Administering appropriate dose, route and type of seizure medication
■ Recognize, anticipate and treat for potential complications of seizure medications
■ Obtain a definitive airway
■ Request and interpret bedside EEG for non-convulsive status epilepticus

Communication and teamwork

■ Obtain accurate history from EMS
■ Recognize difficulty in obtaining history from patient with questionable post-ictal vs. non-convulsive seizure state
■ Work effectively in an interdisciplinary team

3. SUPPLIES

■ IV fluid
■ IO for difficult IV access
■ Syringes for medication administration
■ Non-invasive airway supplies: nasal trumpet, NRB
■ Intubation supplies: BVM, ETT, stylet, blade and handle, suction, back-up airway
■ Medic wrist band for patient with "seizure disorder" written on it

4. MOULAGE

Medic wrist band on a mannequin with seizing functionality.

5. IMAGING AND LABS

■ CT1: normal head CT
■ EKG12: sinus tachycardia
■ Labs: CBC, pregnancy test, blood and urine toxicology

6. ACTORS (CONFEDERATES) AND THEIR ROLES

■ EMS: brings patient to the ED, mentions that patient was initially confused in the ambulance but then seized again and now is no longer responsive in ED; tells team that no medications were given to the patient because they are a BLS ambulance.
■ Nurse: assists the team in following orders, administering medications, etc.
■ Neurology consult (voice): suggests to the team an EEG if not performed, questions the team on performing an LP if it has been performed, recommends definitive airway management if not done; if everything done then the neurologist commends the team and agrees to see patient in the ED.
■ ICU consult (voice): accepts patient to the ICU.

7. CRITICAL ACTIONS

■ Perform thorough neurological exam
■ Recognize convulsive and non-convulsive seizures
■ Administer appropriate medication: dose, route and for type of seizure
■ Secure definitive airway
■ Obtain and interpret EEG accurately
■ Consider LP for patient
■ Obtain neurology consult
■ Admit patient to ICU

8. TIMELINE

Time 0

VS: BP 110/65, HR 110, Sat 97% on 100% O_2, RR 10, 36.4°C, fingerstick glucose 95 (given upon asking)

■ Summary of initial presentation: 31-year-old obese woman is brought in by ambulance by EMS for generalized tonic–clonic seizures as per bystanders. EMS called to coffee shop where witnesses said patient was reading a book, fell to her right side on the chair and started to shake all over and foam at the mouth. Woman was placed on NRB by BLS and transferred to ED. En route, had second seizure lasting 1 minute without return to baseline. Time from onset of first seizure to arrival in the ED was 10 minutes
■ Physical exam
  ▶ General: unresponsive, normocephalic and atraumatic, smells of urine
  ▶ HEENT: Pupils 4 mm equal/reactive

- ▶ Neck: supple
- ▶ Chest: CTAB
- ▶ Heart: regular and tachycardic, no extra heart sounds
- ▶ Abdomen: soft,non-tender,non-distended
- ▶ Skin: no pallor, diaphoresis, cyanosis
- ▶ Neuro: withdrawing to pain symmetrically in upper and lower extremities bilaterally
- ■ Initial interventions: notice Medic wrist band, place patient on the monitor, difficulty getting IV access
- ■ IV placement will take 2 minutes
  - ▶ eventually get 18 G in right AC
  - ▶ central line if requested will take 5 minutes
  - ▶ IO if requested will take 2 minutes
- ■ Hypotension should be treated with normal saline 1 L bolus or more
- ■ EMS: gives the history, states that no medications were given because they were a BLS ambulance, remarks on the smell of the urine, points out the Medic wrist band if the team has not noticed it
- ■ Nurse: assists the team, performs all actions needed

Critical actions
- Place patient on monitor
- Obtain fingerstick glucose
- Perform thorough neurological examination
- Obtain IV access
- Recognize hypotension

Transition point 1: 1 minute

VS: BP 110/65, HR 110, RR 10, Sat 97% on 100% O_2, 36.4°C

- ■ Physical exam: patient with generalized convulsive seizure
  - ▶ third seizure, there is still no IV access
  - ▶ if team gives 5 mg IM midazolam then seizure stops
  - ▶ if team gives PR medication or no IM medication then seizure continues
- ■ If team does not give IV fluid bolus for hypotension, then BP 80/55
- ■ Nurse: assists the team, performs all actions needed

Critical actions
- Treat seizure with midazolam through the IM route
- Attempt venous access through IV, IO or central line method

---

Transition point 2: 3 minutes

VS: BP 80/55 (despite fluid bolus if given), HR 100, RR 6, O_2 Sat 90% on 100% O_2

- ■ Access obtained via IV route
- ■ Physical exam: another generalized convulsive seizure (either a new seizure if stopped the previous minute, or another new seizure)

■ If team gives lorazepam IV ($\geq$10 mg IVP): seizure stops
  ▶ BP 80/55, HR 100, O_2 Sat falls to 90% on 100% O_2, RR falls to 6
■ If lorazepam given as 10 mg divided doses: no hypoxia
  ▶ BP 100/65, HR 90, O_2 Sat 96% on 100% RR 10
■ if lorazepam IV (<10 mg): seizure continues
  ▶ BP 100/65, HR 90 O_2 Sat 96% on 100% O_2, RR 10
■ Nurse points out the change in VSs, gives all medications exactly as ordered

> **Critical actions**
> • Obtain IV access
> • Change seizure medication to lorazepam
> • Recognize side effects of hypotension and respiratory depression

Transition point 3: 4 minutes

VS: BP 100/65, HR 110, RR 8, O_2 Sat 80% on 100% O_2

■ Physical exam: patient with another generalized convulsive seizure (either a new seizure if stopped the previous minute, or another new seizure)
  ▶ if team gives fosphenytoin or phenytoin at 18 mg/kg then seizure stops
  ▶ if team gives fosphenytoin or phenytoin but underdoses then seizure continues
■ VS:
  ▶ if team intubates the patient: BP 100/65, HR 110, Sat 100% on BVM through ETT
  ▶ If team does not intubate the patient: BP 80/50, HR 110, RR 6, O_2 Sat 70% on 100% O_2
■ Nurse: points out the need to intubate the patient if the team does not, suggests the need to give additional medications because of prolonged seizures

> **Critical actions**
> • Give second medication for treatment of status epilepticus
> • Recognize need to intubate the patient because of respiratory depression and because of status epilepticus

Transition point 4: 6 minutes

VS:

■ ▶ if with ETT: BP 100/65, HR 110, Sat 100% on BVM
  ▶ if not intubated: BP 60/30, HR 40, O_2 Sat 50% on 100% O_2, RR 6
■ Physical exam, seizure continues: will need third agent and intubation if not already intubated
■ If pentobarbital (5 mg/kg) given without fluids, will drop pressure
■ Seizures stop with the phenobarbital
■ Nurse: states she notices that the eyes are deviating towards the left
■ If patient not intubated, will go into PEA arrest

Critical actions
- Give third medication for treatment of status epilepticus
- Recognize need to intubate the patient because of respiratory depression and because of status epilepticus

Transition point 5: final actions

VS: if intubated BP 100/65, HR 110, O_2 Sat 100% BVM through ETT

- If PEA arrest: BP 60/30, O_2 Sat 30%
- If intubated: results given of head CT normal, labs with subtherapeutic phenytoin, toxicology screen positive for benzodiazepines, EKG
- Neurology consult: discusses case with the team, should recommend EEG if not done by team
- ICU consult: accepts patient into the ICU
- If PEA, then patient codes until the end of the case

Critical actions
- Recognize importance of EEG in non-convulsive seizures
- Obtain appropriate consult
- Dispose in appropriate setting

9. STIMULI

- CT1: normal head CT
- EKG12: sinus tachycardia
- Labs
  - CBC: WBC 14, Hgb 13.8, hematocrit 34, platelets 150
  - BMP: sodium 132, potassium 7.2, chloride 103, bicarbonate 20, BUN 13, creatinine 9.0, glucose 200, calcium 9.3
  - Urine pregnancy: negative
  - phenytoin: 5
  - valproate acid: undetectable
  - phenobarbital: undetectable
  - urine toxicology: positive for benzodiazepines

10. BIBLIOGRAPHY

ACEP Clinical Policies Subcommittee on Seizures. Clinical policy: critical issues in the evaluation and management of adult patients presenting to the emergency department with seizures. *Ann Emerg Med* 2004; 43:605–25.

Hirsch LJ. Intramuscular versus intravenous benzodiazepines for prehospital treatment of status epilepticus. *N Engl J Med* 2012; 366:659–60.

Prasad K, Al-Roomi K, Krishnan PR, Sequeira R. Anticonvulsant therapy for status epilepticus. *Cochrane Database Syst Rev* 2009; (4):CD00372321

CASE 25

Intracranial hemorrhage

Nikita K. Joshi and Yasuharu Okuda

1. SCENARIO OVERVIEW

A 64-year-old man with history of arrhythmia and hypertension comes to ED with moderate headache, dizziness and numerous episodes of vomiting over 1 hour. Was driven to ED by wife who had to have security carry patient in from car using wheelchair. He had just come home from warfarin clinic when symptoms started. Man denies blurry vision, fever and weakness of arms or legs. Appears mildly agitated and anxious. CT head shows hemorrhagic stroke in cerebellum. Patient gets obtunded after CT and requires emergency airway, management of hypertensive emergency and reversal of supratherapeutic INR.

2. TEACHING OBJECTIVES/DISCUSSION POINTS

Clinical and medical management

■ Activation of stroke code for possible TPA administration
■ Obtaining rapid fingerstick glucose
■ Management of BP with intracranial hemorrhage
■ Reversal of elevated INR
■ Obtaining emergent neurosurgery consult
■ Securing advanced airway

Communication and teamwork

■ Maintaining crowd control
■ Delivering bad news to the wife
■ Reassessment of critically ill patient

3. SUPPLIES

■ Wheelchair
■ IV fluid
■ Syringes with medications
■ Non-invasive airway supplies: nasal trumpet, NRB
■ Intubation supplies: BVM, ETT, stylet, blade and handle, suction, back-up airway

4. MOULAGE

Vomit on the mannequin and bruises on the extremities.

5. IMAGES AND LABS

■ CT6: cerebellar hemorrhage
■ EKG10: rate-controlled atrial fibrillation
■ Labs: CBC, BMP, clotting

6. ACTORS

■ Patient: actor, becomes mannequin after returning from the first head CT.
■ Wife: frantic upset from the vomiting and lacks medical knowledge.
■ Security: helps the wife bring the patient from the parking lot to the ED.
■ Nurse: assists the team with administration and execution of orders.
■ Neurology consult (voice): discusses management with team, recommends a second head CT if not performed.
■ Neurosurgery consult (voice): sounds bored, states no neurosurgical intervention recommended, refuses to come bedside.

7. CRITICAL ACTIONS

■ Activate stroke code for possible TPA administration
■ Obtaining rapid fingerstick glucose
■ Manage BP in intracranial hemorrhage
■ Reverse elevated INR
■ Obtain emergency neurosurgery consult
■ Secure advanced airway

8. TIMELINE

Time 0

VS: BP 220/120, HR 20, RR 90, O_2 Sat 100%, 37.4°C (tympanic), fingerstick glucose 110 (must ask), EKG – rate-controlled atrial fibrillation at 90

■ Summary of initial presentation: 64-year-old man with history of arrhythmia and hypertension comes to ED with moderate headache, dizziness and numerous episodes of vomiting over 1 hour. Was driven to ED by wife and needed wheelchair to get to ED. As per wife had just come home from warfarin clinic when symptoms started
■ Physical exam
  ▶ General: agitated and anxious; in distress secondary to dizziness and vomiting; has repeated episodes of dry heaves; Orientated x3, eyes closed and holding head with hands
  ▶ HEENT: pupils 2 mm equal/reactive, + vertical nystagmus
  ▶ Neck: supple
  ▶ Chest: CTAB
  ▶ Heart: regular rate and rhythm, no extra heart sounds

- ▶ Abdomen: soft, non-tender, non-distended
- ▶ Skin: mild diaphoresis, no cyanosis, no pallor
- ▶ Neuro: difficulty with finger to nose, heal to shin on right, unable to stand
- ◼ Initial intervention
  - ▶ IV placement 18 G in arm; unable to get labs immediately
  - ▶ Place on cardiac monitor
  - ▶ Team should call stroke code for patient with possible cerebellar stroke
  - ▶ EKG present to the team
- ◼ Security: tells team that he had to assist the patient into the wheelchair at the car and that the patient does not look good at all
- ◼ Wife: very upset, crying; states that everything was fine until he came back from the warfarin clinic. She thinks that the patient is on warfarin because of an abnormal heart rhythm. She does not understand why the patient cannot stop vomiting
- ◼ Nurse: helpful and assists the team

Critical actions
- Obtain fingerstick glucose in unstable patient
- Perform thorough neurological physical examination
- Recognize symptoms of cerebellar stroke and call stroke code
- Obtain history of warfarin use

Transition point 1: 2 minutes

VS: BP 220/120, HR 20, RR 90, O$_2$ Sat 100%, EKG – rate-controlled atrial fibrillation at 90

- ◼ Physical exam: unchanged, patient continues to vomit and dry heave
- ◼ If team called a stroke code, then CT calls for patient and states that they are ready for patient
- ◼ Patient gets rolled away on the stretcher with the assistance of the nurse to the CT
- ◼ Wife: very upset, but consolable by the team
- ◼ If stroke code placed: neurology consult calls on the phone and asks for a description of the neurological exam, recommends a stat head CT and recommends stat INR level
- ◼ Nurse: sends off blood work requested by the team and assists in rolling the patient out of the room and switching the actor to the mannequin on the stretcher

Critical actions
- Send off labs appropriate for a stroke code: CBC, CMP, PT/PTT, type and screen
- Stabilize patient to send to CT

Transition point 2: 4 minutes

VS: BP 230/120, HR 10, RR 65, O$_2$ Sat 97%

- ◼ Patient returns from CT as mannequin
- ◼ Physical exam after returning from CT:
  - ▶ General: confused and lethargic
  - ▶ HEENT: pupils 4 mm sluggish, symmetric
  - ▶ Neuro: decorticate posturing

- Head CT images showing cerebellar infarct is presented to team
- Lab calls with stat INR results for stroke code: INR is 4
- Team should recognize need to obtain definitive airway and intubate patient
- Team should obtain stat neurology consult and neurosurgery consult
- Patient lethargic, not following commands, decorticate posturing
- Wife: very upset, agrees to intubation if asked by team
- Nurse: helpful with assisting the team

Critical actions
- Recognize decompensation of patient
- Obtain definitive airway
- Recognize intracranial hemorrhage from supratherapeutic INR
- Recognize hypertensive emergency

Transition point 3: 6 minutes

VS: BP 230/120, HR 10, RR 65, O_2 Sat 97%

- Physical exam
  - General: intubated, sedated, paralyzed
  - HEENT: pupils 4 mm paralyzed
  - Neuro: decorticate posturing
- Team must recognize hypertensive emergency
  - if given nitroglycerin: hypotensive (BP 130/90)
  - if give nitroprusside >1 microg/kg becomes hypotensive (BP 130/90); if given 0.25 microg/kg slowly decreases BP
  - if given labetalol: continues to be hypertensive
  - if given nicardipine (1.2 mg/h): slowly decreases BP
- Team must recognize supratherapeutic INR and administer reversal agents
  - vitamin K: IV bolus over 20 minutes
  - fresh frozen plasma: must call the blood bank, and will take 4 hours to thaw 4 units
  - prothrombin complex concentrate
- Neurosurgery: calls back for consult for cerebellar bleed; initially says to call neurology; must argue to get someone to come down given size and location of bleed and risk for hernation
- Nurse: assists with all orders given

Critical actions
- Deliver bad news to the wife
- Appropriately disposition the patient to the neurosurgery ICU

Transition point 4: final actions

VS: BP based upon medications given, RR 10, HR 65, O_2 Sat 100%

- Physical exam: unchanged
- Team must deliver bad news to the wife regarding diagnosis and treatment of cerebellar hemorrhage

■ Neurosurgery resident calls back and states that patient should be admitted to neurosurgery ICU
■ Wife: questions team regarding prognosis
■ Nurse: helpful with all orders given by team

9. STIMULI

■ CT6: cerebellar hemorrhage
■ EKG10: rate-controlled atrial fibrillation
■ Labs
  ▶ CBC: WBC 17, Hgb 9, hematocrit 30, platelets 200
  ▶ BMP: sodium 133. potassium 4.2, chloride 108, bicarbonate 23, BUN 15, creatinine 3.0, glucose 140, calcium 9.0
  ▶ INR 8.0

10. BIBLIOGRAPHY

Ansell J, J Hirsh, A Jacobson, M Crowther, G Palareti. Pharmacology and management of the vitamin K antagonists: American College of Chest Physicians Evidence-Based Clinical Practice Guidelines (8th edition). *Chest* 2008; 133:160S–198S.

Fallowfield L and V Jenkins. Communicating sad, bad, and difficult news in medicine. *Lancet* 2004; 24:321–329.

Morgenstern LB, JC Hemphill 3rd, C. Anderson et al. Guidelines for the management of spontaneous intracerebral hemorrhage: a guideline for healthcare professionals from the American Heart Association/American Stroke Association. *Stroke* 2010; 41:2108–2129.

Stroke/health information technology

Nikita K. Joshi and Jacqueline A. Nemer

1. SCENARIO OVERVIEW

A 65-year-old man with hypertension, diabetes, hyperlipidemia and prostate cancer suddenly develops slurred speech, drooling and right-sided weakness while golfing with his wife. Wife delayed calling EMS because she initially believes he had a few too many cocktails at the golf course. Patient arrives in ED via EMS appearing to have had a stroke starting 2 1/2 hours ago. Team must consider and address TPA risks and benefits and discuss these with wife. As 3 hours quickly approaches, nurse is questioning the accuracy of the TPA order and wife is questioning the risks of TPA. Hospital has a stroke team who is unavailable.

2. TEACHING OBJECTIVES/DISCUSSION POINTS

Clinical and medical management

- Perform effective resuscitation of a neurologically critical patient
- Identify acute stroke symptoms
- Demonstrate knowledge of indication of TPA in acute stroke

Communication and teamwork

- Demonstrate effective use of TeamSTEPPS in an interdisciplinary team
- Discuss risk and benefits with family regarding TPA
- Navigate ordering of high-risk medications in a complex health information technology system

3. SUPPLIES

- IV fluid
- Syringes with TPA
- Computer for order entry
- Pyxis to obtain medications
- Non-invasive airway supplies: nasal trumpet, NRB
- Intubation supplies: BVM, ETT, stylet, blade and handle, suction, back-up airway

- Phone hang up sound
- Phone "hold" music

4. MOULAGE

- Fluid to mimic drool
- Nurse: white coat
- Wife: head scarf, sunglasses, golf attire
- Patient: golfer hat, sunglasses, golf attire
- Golfer friends: golfer hats, wacky shirts, sunglasses

5. IMAGES AND LABS

- CT1: normal head CT
- EKG1: sinus tachycardia
- Labs: CBC, BMP, clotting, type and screen

6. ACTORS

- Patient: real actor on stretcher who has right facial droop, is drooling, has mild slurred speech, right upper extremity weakness, does not comply with cerebellar exams.
- Mannequin: becomes the patient 1–2 minutes into the case when actor/patient declines from initially mumbling recognizable words to muttering incomprehensible sounds, drooling, grunting/snoring.
- Nurse: insistent upon clarity of all orders prior to execution and upon closed-loop communication.
- Wife: demands team communicates with her every step, anxious about TPA risks, but considered about the delay in administration.
- EMS: gives brief communication of timeline of symptoms.
- Golfer (1 or 2): arrives during case, disruptive and clueless, keeps rambling until dismissed by team.
- Neuro/stroke consult (by phone only): wants concise presentation, too busy with sick patient to come to ED, tells the team to "do the right thing;" calls back at end of case for presentation, asks about wife's reaction to TPA if team did not mention the conflict.
- PMD: (by phone only): "I only have a few minutes" somewhat arrogant, questions team about their TPA decision.

7. CRITICAL ACTIONS

- Perform primary and secondary survey, and full neurological exam
- Request fingerstick glucose
- Obtain stat head CT
- Assess TPA benefits, contraindications and risks for this patient: includes data gathering: contacting the man's personal medical doctor (PMD) for recent labs, PMH, and TPA contraindications
- Discuss TPA consent and TPA risks–benefits with wife

■ Order appropriate TPA dosing in a complex computerized system
■ Case presentation to neurologist attending, including wife's apprehension with
TPA risks

8. TIMELINE

Time 0

VS: BP 200/103, HR 102, RR 20, O$_2$ Sat 98% RA, 37°C, GCS 15, fingerstick glucose 107
(given when asked for); EKG – sinus tachycardia at 105

■ Summary of initial presentation: 65-year-old man PMH hypertension, diabetes,
hyperlipidemia, prostate cancer in remission. Patient and wife were playing golf
when he suddenly develops slurred speech, drooling, and right sided weakness.
Wife delays calling EMS because she initially believes he had a few too many
cocktails at the golf course. Patient arrives in ED via EMS and appears to have a
stroke starting 2 1/2 hours ago
■ Initial intervention: EMS placed IV on left arm
■ Physical exam (patient currently the actor):
  ▶ General: alert, mild confusion, slurred speech, orientated for person/time (not
    place, forgets he is in Denver)
  ▶ Heart: mildly tachycardia, no murmurs
  ▶ Chest: CTAB
  ▶ Abdomen: soft, non-tender, non-distended
  ▶ Neuro: gag intact, when tested patient coughs "hey stop that;" right eye devi-
    ation, right-sided facial droop; drooling, slurred speech; right upper extremity
    weakness, unable to comply with finger to nose
■ EMS: offers brief exam findings of the right-sided weakness and drooling then
quickly exits
■ Wife: anxious; wants to be informed of each step that the doctors are performing;
initially says that the symptoms must only be from the afternoon cocktails, offers
PMD's phone number
■ Nurse: helpful, but insists on clear communication; helps to place patient on the
monitor and begins to obtain bloods

Critical actions
- Primary and secondary survey
- Full neurological examination
- Obtaining fingerstick glucose
- Obtaining full debrief from EMS
- Communicate with the wife

Transition point 1–2 minutes

VS: BP 200/100, HR 100, RR 20, O$_2$ Sat 98% RA

■ Changes in physical exam: GCS 13 (stops responding to commands)
  ▶ If stroke code is called, then patient will go to CT scanner and be replaced with
    mannequin upon return
  ▶ If labetalol 20–40 mg IVP is given, then BP is 170/90

■ Stroke attending clinician: calls back stating he cannot come to code because of another sick patient
■ Patient returns from the CT scanner as the mannequin. He has drooling and sounds of obstructed airway that resolve with jaw thrust; if team assesses airway, patient coughs and states "stop that!"
■ Wife; very nervous and requests specific details about each TPA risk and likelihood in her husband's case, questions if his prostate cancer plays a role, refuses to let the team intubate the patient if the team attempts this:
  ▶ "He drools like this when he's tired after he's had a few cocktails, then he naps"
  ▶ gives consent for TPA "I guess you doctors know better than me"
  ▶ does not know details about patient's medication or PMH, offers PMD's number
■ Nurse: helps with transporting patient out of the room and bringing in mannequin; ensures proper informed consenting procedures are followed

Critical actions
- Initiation of stroke code
- Obtaining fingerstick glucose prior to obtaining head CT
- Timely Brain CT
- Treating elevated BP with labetalol
- Obtaining informed consent from wife
- Effectively working with nurse using TeamSTEPPS methods

Transition point 2: 4 minutes

VS: BP 170/90 (if labetalol given), 200/110 (if no labetalol), HR 100, RR 20, O$_2$ Sat 99% RA, GCS 10

■ Changes in physical exam: Coughing and choking on drool, not opening eyes spontaneously, not speaking legibly
■ Head CT results come back (CT1): display images sequentially
■ Labs available
■ EKG available (EKG1, sinus tachycardia)
■ If team requests to speak to PMD, PMD contacted:
  ▶ arrogant, "blood work done 1 week ago that showed normal platelets and normal creatinine
  ▶ "PMH: prostate cancer 10 years ago"
  ▶ questions TPA, asks if the team are neurologists, questions TPA risks
  ▶ asks to speak with wife, "Are you sure you want him to get this TPA? He's better off now than bleeding into his brain or dead. Good luck with your decision. Got to go"
■ Patient's airway: gag reflex intact; when patient is gagged/vomits or says "stop that!"

Critical actions
- Brain CT interpretation
- Reassess the patient's neurological status and airway; consider intubation
- Obtain key information from PMD
- Interpret labs and EKG
- Communicate effectively with wife and nurse

Transition point 3: 6 minutes

VS: BP 160/90, HR 90, RR 20, O$_2$ Sat 99% RA, GCS 10

- No change in physical exam
- TPA is ordered (0.9 mg/kg; maximum 90 mg over 60 minutes, 10% given as initial IV bolus over 1 minute)
- Nurse: confused over the order and demands clarity
  - ▶ "Pyxis [computer ordering system] won't allow dose TPA since patient weight isn't entered"
  - ▶ confused by the computer and does not understand how the infusion is over 60 minutes, but 10% goes over in the 1 minute; "The computer says to give 90 mg over 1 minute, and then 90 mg more over 60 minutes, but that sounds wrong"
  - ▶ insists on reviewng the step by step calculations with the team and before administering TPA to check the computer system
- Wife: upset by delay since team had stressed the importance of timing, and questions her TPA consent; Eventually agrees to TPA but states she will hold team accountable if husband has bad outcome due to delayed administration
- Golfer(s) return:
  - ▶ question team "How's he doing? What happened?"
  - ▶ when asked about their relationship with patient, say "Just met the couple, but they seemed real nice and just wanted to see how they are doing;" keeps rambling until dismissed by team

---

Critical actions
- Accurately order and administer TPA
- Navigation of difficult ordering system with complex health information technology
- Understand importance of weight-based dosing for TPA
- Removal of unnecessary people, patient privacy

Transition point 4: final actions

VS: BP 160/90, HR 90, RR 20, O$_2$ Sat 99% RA, GCS 10

- No change in physical exam: gag reflex is intact when tested
- TPA is administered once clarity over the order has been achieved and the nurse and team review computer calculations
- Nurse: states her frustration with Pyxis, the computer ordering system, and the team, and voices her concerns about potential bad outcomes from the TPA administration
- PMD: calls back, "Is the TPA in? I just want to be really clear that I had no part of the TPA decision. I don't rush into a big decision like that without a family meeting..." (keeps rambling about his 30+ years in practice until team ends call)
- Neuro/stroke attending clinician: calls and asks team to present case
  - ▶ asks about wife's reaction to TPA if team did not mention the conflict
  - ▶ accepts patient to the neurosurgery ICU

Critical actions
- Effective communication with the wife, nurse, and PMD.
- Give case report to neurologist: situation, background, assessment, recommendation

9. STIMULI

■ CT1: normal head CT
■ EKG1: sinus tachycardia
■ Labs:
  ▶ CBC: WBC 13, Hgb 9, hematocrit 30, platelets 200
  ▶ BMP: sodium 133. potassium 4.2, chloride 108, bicarbonate 23, BUN 15, creatinine 2.3, glucose 140, calcium 9.0
  ▶ PT/PTT: 12/33
  ▶ type and screen

10. BIBLIOGRAPHY

Capella J, Smith S, Philp A, et al. Teamwork training improves the clinical care of trauma patients. *J Surg Educ* 2010; 67:439–43.

Hacke W, Donnan G, Fieschi C, for the ATLANTIS Trials Investigators, ECASS Trials Investigators and NINDS rt-PA Study Group Investigators. Association of outcome with early stroke treatment: pooled analysis of ATLANTIS, ECASS, and NINDS rt-PA stroke trials. *Lancet* 2004;363:768–74.

National Institute of Neurological Disorders and Stroke rt-PA Stroke Study Group. Tissue plasminogen activator for acute ischemic stroke. *N Engl J Med* 1995; 333:1581–7.

Football injury: cervical spine fracture with neurogenic shock

Jacqueline A. Nemer and Marianne Juarez

1. SCENARIO OVERVIEW

A 17-year-old quarterback brought in by ambulance after being tackled and "dog-piled" by multiple players during a playoff game. He was found supine on the bottom of the pile, talking but with confused speech and was carried off the playing field by the sideline athletic trainers and orthopedist. EMTs noted repetitive questioning and confused comments. The event occurred 5 minutes prior to arrival to the ED.

Sideline orthopedist arrives and attempts to take over the case from the ED team, focusing on the bones and joints until a team member addresses him and redirects him away from the patient. Patient's neurological status declines requiring intubation, followed by hypotension refractory to blood and pressors. Team must perform trauma assessment, identify and manage cervical fracture with spinal shock and stabilize for transfer to a neurosurgical center.

Receiving hospital ED is a level 3 trauma center but is the closest hospital to the game. It has the following capabilities:

- all emergency ED labs
- portable radiography: chest, c-spine, pelvis
- CT on third floor and down a long hall
- no neurosurgery service
- no trauma service

2. TEACHING OBJECTIVES/DISCUSSION POINTS

Clinical and medical management

- Objective 1: demonstrate a stepwise approach to the evaluation of a trauma patient (ABCDE)
  - ▶ perform neurological exam prior to administering intubation drugs
  - ▶ expose/undress patient to complete the primary survey
- Objective 2: perform the appropriate steps in airway control in a helmeted patient
  - ▶ non-invasive airway control with c-spine immobilization
  - ▶ jaw thrust for suctioning
  - ▶ ± nasal trumpet placement

▶ facemask/pad removal
▶ intubation with attention to c-spine immobilization and suspected closed head injury
■ Objective 3: demonstrate the appropriate initial management of hypotension in a trauma patient
▶ IV access
▶ IV fluid resuscitation
▶ vasopressors as indicated
■ Objective 4: develop differential diagnosis list for traumatic hypotension
▶ hemorrhagic shock: splenic/liver laceration, long bone fractures, etc.
▶ acute blunt cardiac injury
▶ neurogenic shock
■ Objective 5: recognize neurogenic shock and initiate the appropriate initial management
▶ IV fluid resuscitation
▶ vasopressors
▶ consider steroids

Communication and teamwork

■ Objective 1: interprofessional communication with EMT, orthopedist, neurosurgeon and family

3. SUPPLIES

■ Football helmet, shoulder pads, jersey, mouth guard
■ Non-invasive airway equipment
■ Intubation equipment and suction
■ Confederate's clothing:
▶ sports medicine jacket for orthopedist
▶ nursing attire
■ IV administration equipment
■ Mock pints of blood products
■ Mock medications

4. MOULAGE

■ Make-up to create bruising over anterior chest wall and dried blood around lips
■ Family member's team fan's sports attire and foam "1" finger

5. IMAGES AND LABS

■ XR1: normal male CXR
■ XR3: normal male CXR with ETT in correct position
■ XR13: lateral view of C1–C6, cannot visualize C7
■ XR14: odontoid view with C1 Jefferson fracture
■ US1: normal FAST
■ Labs: BMP, CBC, O_2 Sat

6. ACTORS (CONFEDERATES) AND THEIR ROLES

- Patient: simulator.
- Nurse: IV access, medication administration.
- EMT: initial history and exam findings.
- Sideline orthopedic doctor: attempts to run resuscitation initially, obstructive to team until acknowledged and redirected.
- Radiology technician: performs plain films and encourages team to remove helmet/pads prior to imaging, also prompts team to reposition patient inappropriately.
- Neurosurgery consult (phone): prompts team to order any additional tests prior to transfer to a trauma center.
- Family member: available to provide additional PMH 2–3 minutes after case has begun.

7. CRITICAL ACTIONS

- Complete primary survey (ABCDE): disability must be checked prior to giving intubation medication; fully expose patient noting chest wall contusions
- Use appropriate procedure for facemask removal
- Control airway while maintaining c-spine immobilization
- Treat hypotension in a trauma patient (initially order IV fluids and request blood, while considering the differential diagnosis for this)
- Recognize neurogenic shock, order pressors

8. TIMELINE

Time 0

VS: BP 125/80, HR 109, RR 36, O_2 Sat 88% RA, 37.0°C, fingerstick glucose 90 (if requested), EKG – sinus tachycardia

- Summary of initial presentation: 17-year-old man with helmet and shoulder pads on, repetitive questioning, rapid shallow respirations, a small amount of blood on lips and mouth guard, pooling saliva
- Physical exam
  - General: fully dressed in jersey, shoulder pads and helmet
  - HEENT: small amount of blood on mouth guard, + gag reflex
  - Neck: trachea midline, no c-spine step-off palpated, unclear about midline tenderness due to confused speech, "shake it off"
  - Chest: tachypnea, rapid but shallow breathing, bruising over the anterior chest, stable, no crepitus
  - Heart: tachycardia, rate/rhythm regular, no m/r/g
  - Abdomen: soft, without masses, normal bowel sounds, no bruising
  - Rectal: (if performed) weak tone, normal prostate position, no blood
  - Skin: bruising on anterior chest wall
  - Neuro: sleepy but arousable, oriented to name; eyes open to verbal stimuli; verbal response delayed, confused, with slow speech and nonsensical answers such as "got it coach," "shake it off" and repeating team comments; does not

move any extremities spontaneously or withdrawal to pain but patient answers "got it coach" when any extremity is tested; low muscle tone if asked

■ Initial interventions:

▶ IV access: not present upon arrival

▶ EKG: sinus tachycardia 110

■ EMT: provides initial history and field vitals

Critical actions
- Order IV access
- Place on monitor
- Bedside glucose

Transition point 1: 1 minutes

VS: BP 120/80, HR 112, RR 36, O_2 Sat 88% RA 37.0°C

■ ABCD – if patient, then airway assessed, suctioned, $\pm$ nasal trumpet: gag reflex, "Come on Coach"

■ Supplemental O_2 applied:

▶ RR decreases to 30

▶ Increases SO_2 to maximum of 95%

▶ respiratory status remains stable initially giving team time to perform neurological exam prior to intubation

■ IV access ordered:

▶ achieved within 1 minute

▶ serum for labs obtained and sent if ordered

▶ IV fluids started if ordered

■ Labs: none available

■ Imaging: none available

■ Orthopedist: starts out by running the trauma and giving team orders; if addressed/redirected, he remains cooperative and out of the way; if disregarded, he delays the initial ABCs and becomes obstructive

---

Critical actions
- Supplemental O_2 administration for hypoxia
- IV fluid hydration and labs ordered

Transition point 2: 2 minutes

VS: BP 109/68, HR 82, RR 10, O_2 Sat 91% RA

■ Changes in physical exam/condition

▶ General: still in helmet and pads

▶ Chest: breathing more shallow

▶ Neuro: no longer talking, eyes closed, do not open to voice or pain

■ Exposure

▶ facemask removal while maintaining c-spine precautions

▶ pads and helmet removal while maintaining c-spine precautions

■ Labs: none available
■ Imaging:
  ▶ for either c-spine or chest images, radiology technician prompts team to remove pads and helmet prior to imaging as X-ray beam will not penetrate gear
  ▶ if c-spine images ordered prior to helmet/pad removal, radiology technician asks team to pull down arms for better image quality: CRITICAL ERROR if team does this
  ▶ if CXR ordered, radiology technician asks team to move and roll patient to place plate: CRITICAL ERROR if team does this
■ Radiology technician:
  ▶ prompts team to remove gear prior to imaging
  ▶ asks for assistance in obtaining imaging by asking team to pull down arms for c-spine image and move/roll patient for CXR

Transition point 3: 4 minutes

■ Intubation: if team is not preparing for intubation, allow radiography to be performed
  ▶ VS: BP 108/58,, HR 80, RR 10 on 76% NRB
  ▶ c-spine immobilization
  ▶ RSI for suspected head/c-spine-injured patient
  ▶ order post-intubation CXR; if not done, nurse prompts team to do so
■ If team orders CT of head/c-spine, nurse informs that closest scanner is on third floor, encourages portable c-spine radiography
■ Labs: VBG, lactate
■ Imaging:
  ▶ post-intubation CXR (XR3)
  ▶ FAST if ordered (US1): normal
■ Nurse: prompts team to obtain portable imaging if requesting CT scan and prompts for post-intubation CXR if not ordered

---

Critical actions
- Intubate
- Order post-intubation CXR
- Order c-spine imaging

Transition point 4: 6 minutes

■ Post-intubation hypotension
  ▶ VS: BP 78/43, HR 45, O_2 Sat 100% intubated
  ▶ volume resuscitation with IV fluid ± blood transfusion order
  ▶ EKG: sinus bradycardia (EKG5)
■ Family member: arrives; hysterical and must be counseled or will become obstructive
■ Imaging:
  ▶ XR13: lateral view C1–C6 with no obvious fracture, cannot assess C7
  ▶ XR14: odontoid view with C1 Jefferson fracture

■ Radiologist: calls with wet read "possible unstable C1 fracture, correlate clinically" if team does not recognize fracture
■ Vasopressor ordered ± steroid
■ Nurse: prompts if not ordered "Blood pressure not responding to IV fluid hydration and blood transfusion"
■ Neurosurgery paged

Critical actions
- Volume resuscitate
- Recognize c-spine injury
- Recognize neurogenic shock
- Order vasopressor(s) ± steroids

Transition point 4: final actions

■ Response to vasopressor(s)
  ▶ if ordered, BP 100/70, HR 92
  ▶ if not ordered, BP 60/35, HR 45
■ Neurosurgery surgeon: asks team for clarification of the aspects of trauma work-up still pending and requests the necessary remaining tests and procedures prior to transfer to a trauma center
■ Team must decide in which order to obtain the following:
  ▶ head, chest, abdomen/pelvis CT scans
  ▶ sedation
  ▶ additional vasopressor orders
  ▶ Foley catheter placement
  ▶ NG tube placement
■ Family member: must be informed of c-spine injury and the need for transfer to a trauma center
■ Disposition: transfer to trauma center

Critical actions
- Presentation to neurosurgeon
- Inform family member of injury and disposition
- Appropriate work-up/stabilization prior to transfer

9. STIMULI

■ XR1: normal male CXR
■ XR2: female CXR
■ XR13: lateral view of C1–C6, cannot visualize C7
■ XR14: odontoid view with C1 Jefferson fracture
■ US1: normal FAST
■ EKG5: sinus bradycardia
■ Labs:

BMP	
Sodium	140 mEq/L
Potassium	4.0 mEq/L
Chloride	100 mEq/L
Bicarbonate	22 mEq/L
BUN	14 mg/dL
Creatinine	0.9 mg/dL
Glucose	90 mg/dL
WBC	13 700/mm^3
Hgb	14 g/dL
Hematocrit	44%
Platelets	450/mm^3
Lactate	1.9 mmol/L
O$_2$ Sat	
pH	7.48
PaCO$_2$	25 mmHg
PaO$_2$	66 mmHg
O$_2$ Sat (FiO$_2$ 0.21)	84%

10. BIBLIOGRAPHY

Baron BJ, McSherry KJ, Larson JL, Jr., Scalea TM. Spine and spinal cord trauma. In Tintinalli JE, Stapczynski JS, Cline DM et al. eds. *Tintinalli's Emergency Medicine: A Comprehensive Study Guide*, 7th edn. New York: McGraw-Hill, 2011, Ch. 255.

Mower WR, Hoffman JR, Mahadevan SV. Cervical spine fractures. In Wolfson AB, Hendey GW, Ling LJ et al. eds. *Harwood-Nuss' Clinical Practice of Emergency Medicine*, 5th edn. Philadelphia, PA: Lippincott Williams & Wilkins, 2010, Ch. 28.

Waninger KN. Management of the helmeted athlete with suspected cervical spine injury. *Am J Sports Med* 2004; 32:1331–50.

SECTION 6

OBSTETRICS/ GYNECOLOGY

Floppy newborn resuscitation

Christopher G. Strother

1. SCENARIO OVERVIEW

A 32-week premature infant is born to a pre-eclamptic mother in the resuscitation area. The infant is born blue, floppy and apneic. The team must use good NALS principles to revive the infant. If good-quality CPR is done the infant will slowly improve but will relapse with any poor resuscitation or post-resuscitation care (i.e. inadequate warming).

2. TEACHING OBJECTIVES/DISCUSSION POINTS

Clinical and medical management

■ Chest compressions for newborns with heart rates less than 60 bpm
■ BVM for newborns with heart rates less than 100 bpm
■ Warmth is essential in newborns and hypothermia can lead quickly to deterioration

Communication and teamwork

■ Team leader should have an overview and not be directly involved in procedures
■ Communication of changing vital signs on exam between members and to leader is essential

3. SUPPLIES

■ Newborn simulator, umbilical pulse is ideal
■ Newborn BVM
■ Warmer, blankets

4. MOULAGE

Vernix: a mixture of 100% silicone, baby powder and water can be used.

5. IMAGES AND LABS

None.

6. ACTORS (CONFEDERATES) AND THEIR ROLES

■ Patient: mannequin only.
■ Nurse: can point out mistakes ("Shouldn't you put him under the warmer?").
■ NICU consult: can be consulted for admission but will not be helpful, "We'll come down in a bit."
■ Mother of baby: just delivered, can be a second patient to manage or just asking questions.

7. CRITICAL ACTIONS

■ Recognize severe bradycardia and start good infant CPR
■ Recognize moderate bradycardia and continue BVM when HR is >60
■ Keep the infant warm and dry, and stimulate
■ Infant must be placed under a warmer as fast as possible and kept there

8. TIMELINE

Time 0 (apnea and bradycardia)

VS: HR 40, RR 0, 34.0°C (skin probe), rhythm on monitor not available, vernix will not allow lead placement

■ Summary of initial presentation: blue, floppy, apneic newborn infant; cool to touch, vernix covered (± meconium)
■ Initial interventions: handed directly from obstetrics to team
■ Physical exam
   ▶ General: blue, cold, floppy, apneic
   ▶ HEENT: normal
   ▶ Lungs: coarse when ventilated, apneic
   ▶ Heart: S1S2, no m/r/g, bradycardic
   ▶ Abdomen: normal, normal three-vessel cord
   ▶ Extremities: cyanotic
■ Parents: ask questions

Critical actions
- Warm, dry, stimulate
- Suction briefly
- Feel pulse, note bradycardia and start CPR
- Good compressions and BVM (3:1 ratio)

Transition point 1: 2 minutes (improved if CPR)

VS: HR 75, RR 0

■ Increased HR, still unresponsive
■ If patient received high-quality CPR in the beginning, then HR will be at 70; if not, will remain at 40

▓ Can stop compressions: must continue BVM; if not BVM, HR will return to 40
▓ Labs: none available
▓ Imaging: none available
▓ Parent: asks questions

Critical actions
- Reassess pulse
- Stop CPR, continue BVM
- Continue warmth
- Consider naloxone

Transition point 2: 5 minutes (beginning cry/movement)

VS: HR 120, RR 20

▓ Color improving, beginning to grunt/make noise and move
▓ If patient is not warmed and dried, will again decompensate
▓ Labs: fingerstick glucose 70
▓ Parent: relieved by baby-making noise, want to hold baby
▓ Additional points: as infant begins breathing, warmth and stimulation are key. NICU should be called by now if not already alerted. Other labs and imaging will not be available or needed

Critical actions
- BVM may be stopped when HR >100 and breathing on its own
- Must continue warmth and stimulation

Transition point 3: 7 minutes (stabilization)

VS: HR 140, RR 40

▓ Changes in physical exam/patient condition: increased crying, movement, better color
▓ NICU consult: can accept patient; will not give direct care advice
▓ Parents: need to be informed of progress, future direction for baby's care

Critical actions
- Continued warmth and stimulation/drying
- Consult NICU

Transition point 4: final actions

VS: as above

▓ Changes in physical exam: none
▓ NICU consult: call if not already called

■ Additional points: remember at no point in this resuscitation is an IV/UV/IO line needed. Labs except glucose are not needed nor helpful in initial infant resuscitation. Teams should not rush to intubate as BVM is generally easy and all that is necessary

■ Disposition: NICU

Critical actions
- Wrap/cover infant

9. STIMULI

None.

10. BIBLIOGRAPHY

American Heart Association and American Academy of Pediatrics. 2005 American Heart Association (AHA) guidelines for cardiopulmonary resuscitation (CPR) and emergency cardiovascular care (ECC) of pediatric and neonatal patients: neonatal resuscitation guidelines. *Pediatrics* 2006; 117:e978–e988.

Biban P, Filipovic-Grcic B, Biarent D et al. New cardiopulmonary resuscitation guidelines 2010: managing the newly born in the delivery room. *Early Hum Dev* 2011; 87(Suppl 1): S9–S11.

Kattwinkel J, Perlman JM, Aziz K et al. Part 15: neonatal resuscitation: 2010 American Heart Association Guidelines for Cardiopulmonary Resuscitation and Emergency Cardiovascular Care. *Circulation* 2010; 122:S909–S919.

Roehr CC, Hansmann G, Hoehn T, Buhrer C. The 2010 Guidelines on Neonatal Resuscitation (AHA, ERC, ILCOR): similarities and differences – what progress has been made since 2005? *Klin Padiatr* 2011; 223:299–307.

Postmortem cesarean section with seizing neonate at delivery

Nicholas Renz, Christopher Sampson and Jason Wagner

1. SCENARIO OVERVIEW

A 32-year-old woman with a history of pre-eclampsia G1P0 at 38 weeks arrives via EMS. EMS called to home for seizure. Patient post-ictal on their arrival but during transport patient had two more seizures followed by cardiac arrest 3 minutes ago. CPR in progress on arrival.

2. TEACHING OBJECTIVES/DISCUSSION POINTS

Clinical and medical management

- Objective 1: understand the indications for perimortem cesarean section (C-section)
  - infant viability (>24 weeks or fundal height above the umbilicus)
  - fetal outcome is best if C-section performed within 5 minutes of maternal arrest
  - continue maternal CPR and resuscitation efforts throughout delivery
  - place patient in left lateral decubitus position with towels during CPR
- Objective 2: know appropriate neonatal resuscitation for newborn with seizure
  - airway support
  - consider hypoglycemia: Accucheck/D10 infusion
  - consider electrolyte abnormalities
  - consider infection
  - most common cause is HIE (hypoxic–ischemic encephalopathy)
  - appropriate use of antiepileptics

Communication and teamwork

- Objective 1: team needs to initially focus on maternal resuscitation and evaluation
- Objective 2: early decision for perimortem C-section is essential
- Objective 3: team is required to divide up and prepare for the eventuality of caring for two patients after delivery and be prepared for neonatal resuscitation; roles need to be assigned appropriately for C-section, maternal resuscitation and neonatal resuscitation

3. SUPPLIES

- Female simulator
- Neonatal simulator
- C-section tray
- OHIO table and neonatal resuscitation supplies (airway, umbilical line, medication, etc.)
- Cord clamp
- Perimortem C-section model as described elsewhere attached to female simulator (described in Sampson et al.)

4. MOULAGE

None.

5. IMAGES AND LABS

- US5: fetal heart indicating viability
- Newborn accucheck result
- US6: maternal cardiac arrest
- Labs: glucose

6. ACTORS (CONFEDERATES) AND THEIR ROLES

- Patient: young female mannequin.
- EMS: brings patient into ED and provide HPI as listed above, performing CPR and ventilating by BVM on arrival.
- Consult: NICU accepts newborn.
- Father: upset and requires consultation and explanation of the actions performed by the team during the scenario.

7. CRITICAL ACTIONS

- Focus on maternal resuscitation initially with attention to airway (advanced airway is optional, supraglottic should at least be placed), CPR and place patient in left lateral decubitus position to improve venous return; use IV fluids and code medication as indicated
- Perform C-section immediately on arrival of patient (checking fetal heart viability is optional)
- Check APGAR score in infant
- Check blood glucose on seizing neonate
- Administer dextrose-10 to correct hypoglycemia
- Admit infant to NICU
- Console and discuss with father

8. TIMELINE

Time 0

VS: BP NA, HR NA, RR 16 by BVM, O_2 Sat 100%, 36.5°C, EKG – asystole

- Summary of initial presentation: 32-year-old pregnant woman arrives in cardiac arrest with CPR in progress

- Initial interventions:
  - 18-gauge peripheral IV placed by EMS
  - CPR in progress
  - BVM ventilation
- Physical exam
  - General: unresponsive pregnant woman at term
  - HEENT: clear, BVM ventilation in progress, pupils fixed and dilated
  - Chest: lungs clear to auscultation with bagging
  - Cardiac: CPR in progress
  - Abdomen: term gravid uterus
  - Skin: warm
  - Neuro: unresponsive
- Father/husband: upset and wants to know what is going on

Critical actions
- Place supraglottic airway
- Continue CPR
- Place mother in left lateral decubitus position
- Decision and preparations for perimortem C-section

Transition point 1: 2 minutes

VS: unchanged

- Changes in physical exam: none
- If no actions to perform C-section taken, then father should inquire if the baby is alright
  - Labs: maternal glucose 95
- Imaging:
  - US6: maternal cardiac arrest
  - US5: fetal heart indicating viability

Critical actions
- C-section should be underway at this point
- Continued efforts toward maternal resuscitation including CPR, ventilation, IV normal saline and code medication as indicated
- Roles should be assigned to (a) maternal resuscitation, (b) c-section delivery, (c) neonatal resuscitation

---

Transition point 2: 3 minutes

Mother
VS: unchanged

- Changes in physical exam/condition: none
- Labs: NA
- Imaging: continued maternal cardiac standstill on ultrasound and asystole on monitor
- Father: very anxious about what is happening in front of him

Infant
VS: BP NA, HR 80, pulse oximetry not detecting initially

■ Physical exam (APGAR):
  ▶ appearance: bluish
  ▶ pulse <100
  ▶ grimace: weak cry when stimulated
  ▶ activity: some flexion with stimulation
  ▶ respiration: weak
■ Labs: Accucheck is 20 if requested
■ Imaging: none available
■ Additional points: APGAR improves slightly with oxygenation and stimulation

Critical actions
- Rapid C-section, delivery of infant, cord clamped and cut; hand over to neonatal resuscitation team
- Ongoing maternal CPR
- Team prepared with OHIO table and resuscitation equipment ready
- Neonate resuscitation team notes low APGAR score and makes appropriate efforts toward drying, stimulation, O$_2$ation and reassessment

Transition point 3: 6 minutes

Mother
VS: no change

Infant
VS: BP NA, HR 75, HR 10%, pulse oximetry 98%

■ Changes in physical exam/patient condition: begins turning head to the side and exhibits clonus followed by violent shaking of limbs if hypoglycemia is not detected by this time
■ Labs: Accucheck is 20 if requested
■ Father: identifies seizure-like activity of infant if not noted by resuscitation team "It looks like he's having a seizure"
■ Additional points
  ▶ if hypoglycemia was identified and treated appropriately the infant continues to improve, does not require intubation and has 5-minute APGAR of 9
  ▶ if hypoglycemia is not identified, the infant goes into cardiac arrest within 2 minutes of seizure and will not respond to any treatment other than glucose

Critical actions
- Rapid identification and treatment of hypoglycemia with dextrose-10 in water (D10W)
- Obtain umbilical venous access for administration of dextrose

Transition point 4: final actions

Mother
Despite ongoing resuscitative efforts, ROSC is not obtained; pupils are fixed and dilated and there is asystole on the monitor and cardiac standstill on bedside ultrasound.

Infant
If not treated for hypoglycemia, is in asystole and simulation should be stopped at this time.

If treated with dextrose in timely fashion, VS: HR 130, HR 25, pulse oximetry 100%

- ■ Changes in physical exam (APGAR)
  - ▶ appearance: pink throughout
  - ▶ pulse >100
  - ▶ grimace: strong cry when stimulated
  - ▶ activity: active movement
  - ▶ respiration: spontaneous and regular
- ■ Father: tearful and enquiring about mother and infant
- ■ Disposition: infant to NICU, mother to morgue for autopsy

Critical actions
- • Infant is appropriately resuscitated and NICU consultant accepts infant to NICU
- • Mother is declared deceased after appropriate interventions are exhausted
- • Father/husband is updated and consoled

9. STIMULI

- ■ US6: maternal cardiac arrest, cardiac standstill throughout
- ■ US5: fetal heart indicating viability
- ■ Maternal glucose 95
- ■ Initial fetal glucose 25

10. BIBLIOGRAPHY

American College of Obstetricians and Gynecologists. *ACOG Educational Bulletin 249: Obstetric Aspects of Trauma Management*. Washington DC: American College of Obstetricians and Gynecologists, 1998.

American College of Obstetricians and Gynecologists. *ACOG Practice Bulletin 100: Critical Care in Pregnancy*. Washington DC: American College of Obstetricians and Gynecologists, 2009.

Katz VL, Dotters DJ, Droegenmueller W. Perimortem cesarean delivery. *Obstet Gynecol* 1986; 63:571–576.

McGowan, JE. Neonatal hypoglycemia. *Pediatric Rev* 1999; 20:e6–e15.

Sampson C, Renz NR, Wagner J. An inexpensive and novel model for perimortem cesarean section. *Simul Healthc* 2013; 8:49–51.

Shoulder dystocia with postpartum hemorrhage

Jason Wagner, Christopher Sampson and Brian Bausano

1. SCENARIO OVERVIEW

A 28-year-old woman G3P2 at approximately 38 weeks of pregnancy presents to ED. She has received no prenatal care but states her last baby was "big." Her water broke about 1 hour prior to arrival and contractions are less than 2 minutes apart. Patient presents in active labor pushing as the case begins. When team inspects vagina they find crowning head with turtle sign (between pushes the fetal head moves back into the vaginal canal). No progression and no obstetrics available. Once team performs maneuvers for shoulder dystocia, baby is delivered in mild distress requiring some resuscitation. Mother has heavy vaginal bleeding requiring fundal massage, oxytocin and transfusion of PRBC.

2. TEACHING OBJECTIVES/DISCUSSION POINTS

Clinical and medical management

■ Recognize shoulder dystocia
■ Perform maneuvers for shoulder dystocia
■ Newborn resuscitation
■ Recognition and treatment of postpartum hemorrhage

Communication and teamwork

■ Teamwork and communication for preparation of mother and infant for delivery
■ Division of team for resuscitation of baby as well as mother
■ Communication with mother and father as to what is happening

3. SUPPLIES

Setup to simulate vaginal delivery.
Suggest: birth model that can simulate dystocia (e.g. Noel or MommaNatalie)

4. MOULAGE

None.

5. IMAGES AND LABS

■ EKG4: fetal heart trace
■ No US available because of the emergency nature of delivery but this could be an optional addition

6. ACTORS (CONFEDERATES) AND THEIR ROLES

■ Patient: delivering mother in moderate distress.
■ Nurse: facilitates needs of team, cooperative.
■ Husband: the bigger the actor the better; happy go-lucky at start of case but becomes increasingly distressed as case progresses; can be obstructionist if team is running away with case.
■ Second nurse (optional): depending on skill level of team may need second nurse for neonatal resuscitation.

7. CRITICAL ACTIONS

■ Recognize impending labor
■ Recognize shoulder dystocia
■ Institute proper maneuvers for shoulder dystocia
  ▶ McRoberts maneuver
  ▶ superpubic pressure
  ▶ delivery of posterior arm
  ▶ scapular pressure
  ▶ delivery within 5 minutes
■ Resuscitate infant
■ Recognize and treat postpartum hemorrhage

8. TIMELINE

Time 0

VS: BP 133/88, HR 103, RR 20, O_2 Sat 99% RA, 37.2°C

■ Summary of initial presentation: mother presents to ED by private vehicle in active labor with immediate urge to push
■ Initial interventions: none
■ Physical exam
  ▶ HEENT: within normal limits
  ▶ Chest: CTAB; no wheezes, rales or rhonchi
  ▶ Heart: regular rate and rhythm; no m/r/g
  ▶ Abdomen: gravid uterus 20 cm above umbilicus
  ▶ Extremities: within normal limits
  ▶ Neuro: grossly intact with no deficits
  ▶ Skin: no rash
  ▶ Genital: crowning head with turtle sign between pushing

◾ Nurse (one or two): cooperative; will assist team to best of their ability but not offer advice
◾ Father: excited and anxious, happy

Critical actions
- Recognize impending delivery
- Preparation for delivery

Transition point 1: 2 minutes

VS: BP 133/88, HR 110, RR 20, O_2 Sat 99% RA

◾ Mother cooperates with pushing but tires out and between pushes the fetal head is noted to move back into the vaginal canal (turtle sign)
◾ If team hooks up to tocodynamometer, show image of late decelerations
◾ Labs: none available
◾ Imaging: tocodynamometer with lateral decelerations
◾ Father: notes that something is not right and is becoming more anxious
◾ Initial maneuver for dystocia fails

Critical actions
- Recognize dystocia
- Perform maneuvers for dystocia
- Call for help

Transition point 2: 5 minutes

VS: BP 133/88, HR 110, RR 20, O_2 Sat 99% RA

◾ Patient continues to push with no progression of delivery
◾ Labs: none available
◾ Imaging: tocodynamometer with late decelerations
◾ Father: becoming increasingly anxious; if team is rapidly progressing through case, he may become obstructionist to slow them down
◾ Delivery is successful after team performs two or three maneuvers for dystocia
◾ Mother has heavy vaginal bleeding immediately following delivery

Critical actions
- Attempt various maneuvers for dystocia
- Preparation for baby
- Delivery of baby

Transition point 3: 6 minutes

Mother
VS: BP 80/55, HR 130, RR 22, O_2 Sat 99% RA

◾ Changes in physical exam/patient condition: increasing hemorrhage and worsening BP until team performs critical actions

Baby
VS: systolic BP 65, HR 130, RR 48, O_2 Sat 85% RA to 99% blow-by

■ Changes in physical exam/patient condition:
▶ APGAR score 8 at 1 minute 8, 10 at 5 minutes
▶ immediately perks up with stimulation, warming, and blow-by O_2

Case progress
■ Father: continues to be anxious; if team is rapidly progressing through case may become obstructionist to slow them down; threatens law suits if baby does not turn out OK
■ Depending on team progress, you may have to decrease or increase the level of chaos created by instability of mother and baby along with the father's antics

Critical actions
● Resuscitate baby
● Uteran massage
● Oxytocin
● Transfuse PRBC

Transition point 4: final actions

Mother
VS: BP 110/75, HR 87, RR 16, O_2 Sat 99% RA

Baby
VS: systolic BP 65, HR 125, RR 40, O_2 Sat 99% RA

■ Physical exam/patient condition: APGAR score 10 at 5 minutes

Completion
■ Neither patient should die due to mismanagement
■ Mother and baby stabilized and more comfortable after resuscitations
■ Father: thanks team for all their help and is much more calm

9. STIMULI

■ EKG4: fetal heart trace

10. BIBLIOGRAPHY

Allen RH. On the mechanical aspects of shoulder dystocia and birth injury. *Clin Obstet Gynecol* 2007; 50:607–23.
Spong CY, Beall M, Rodrigues D, Ross MG. An objective definition of shoulder dystocia: prolonged head-to-body delivery intervals and/or the use of ancillary obstetric maneuvers. *Obstet Gynecol* 1995; 86:433–6.

SECTION 7

PEDIATRICS

Pediatric status epilepticus

Scott Goldberg and Steven A. Godwin

1. SCENARIO OVERVIEW

A 14-month-old child is brought to the ED by his mother. He has had 1 day of fever, nasal congestion and occasional cough. He is febrile and begins to seize. The seizure breaks, but the patient has a second seizure that is difficult to treat. The patient's mother becomes hysterical, creating a challenge in situational control.

2. TEACHING OBJECTIVES/DISCUSSION POINTS

Clinical and medical management

■ Identify the causes and management of fever in a pediatric patient
■ Treat refractory seizure in a pediatric patient
■ Manage respiratory decompensation requiring airway intervention in a pediatric patient

Communication and teamwork

■ Utilize appropriate crew resource management to manage a critically ill pediatric patient
■ Implement de-escalation techniques and situational control
■ Make sound disposition arrangements through consultation with appropriate services

3. SUPPLIES

None.

4. MOULAGE

None.

5. IMAGES AND LABS

Point of care blood glucose. No additional labs or imaging will be available.

6. ACTORS (CONFEDERATES) AND THEIR ROLES

- Nurse: generally helpful; may need to prompt teams on the patient's seizure activity.
- Mother: progressively distraught and obstructionist throughout case; hinders clinical care towards the end of the case.
- PICU: will provide additional management recommendations as needed; will accept the transfer of the patient to the PICU if requested.

7. CRITICAL ACTIONS

- Initiate appropriate initial management of the febrile pediatric patient including antipyretics
- Discuss a differential for pediatric seizure
- Manage respiratory decompensation with ETT
- Start appropriate investigations for complex febrile seizures
- Institute appropriate management for a difficult parent who is obstructing clinical care

8. TIMELINE

Time 0

VS: BP 92/50, HR 185, RR 30, O_2 Sat 99% RA, 41.1°C, EKG – sinus tachycardia

- Summary of initial presentation: 14-month-old boy brought in by mother having had 1 day of fevers, nasal congestion and intermittent cough. No trouble breathing and has not had any abdominal pain, vomiting or diarrhea. He has had decreased appetite and activity
- The child is awake and alert, sitting on his mother's lap
- PMH: full term, no medical problems
- Surgical history: none
- Social history: lives with mother, no daycare
- Medication: none
- Allergies: NKDA
- Immunizations: up to date
- Physical exam
  - General: awake, alert, appears generally unwell
  - HEENT: pupils equal/reactive, oropharynx clear, clear rhinorrhea
  - Neck: supple
  - Chest: clear to auscultation bilaterally
  - Heart: tachycardia, no murmurs
  - Abdomen: soft, non-tender, non-distended, no masses
  - Genitourinary: normal
  - Skin: no rashes, warm to touch
  - Neuro: awake, alert, somewhat decreased activity
- Mother: unconcerned, "His brothers and sisters always get these bugs"

Critical actions
- Primary survey
- Antipyretics
- Thorough history and physical examination

Transition point 1: 1 minute

VS: BP 92/50, HR 185, RR 30, O_2 Sat 92% RA

- Begins seizing at 1 minute regardless of case progression: generalized tonic clonic
- Seizure will break after 30 seconds: prior to administration of any medication
- Blood glucose: 178
- Nurse: may have to prompt team regarding seizure activity or seizure termination
- Mother: increasingly concerned, "What's happening to him?"

Critical actions
- Position patient to maintain airway
- Supplemental O_2
- Check blood glucose
- Attempt IV access
- Consider anticonvulsant/benzodiazepine
- Differential for pediatric seizure

Transition point 2: 2–3 minutes

VS: BP 95/50, HR 170, RR 30, O_2 Sat 88% RA, 92% NC, 97% NRB

- The patient is post-ictal, convulsions having terminated
- After 30 seconds move to next transition
- Mother: progressively concerned, disruptive, trying to get close to and hold child

Critical actions
- Continue investigations including blood work if it has not already been done
- De-escalate mother, scene control

Transition point 3: 3–7 minutes

VS: BP 95/50, HR 180, RR 30, O_2 Sat 80% RA, 84% NC, 88% NRB

- Child is seizing again: generalized tonic-clonic
  - ▶ if benzodiazepines given: no change
  - ▶ if phenytoin/fosphenytoin given: no change
  - ▶ if barbiturate or propofol given: seizure will break
  - ▶ if not intubated, respiratory depression and fall in O_2 saturation
- Mother: progressively disruptive, inconsolable, reaching out for child

> **Critical actions**
> - Seizure should be managed with a combination of agents
> - Airway should be managed via intubation prior to, or concurrent with, barbiturate or propofol administration
> - If RSI is used, a short-acting paralytic should be chosen
> - Mother should be removed from scene

Transition point 4: final actions

VS: BP 90/48, HR 150, on ventilation, O_2 Sat 98% (on ventilation)

■ Patient is calm on the ventilator

■ If a paralytic has been used, there will be no further seizure activity

■ If no paralytic has been used, there will be intermittent short bursts of seizure activity

■ PICU: will accept the patient and will recommend any further management that the team has not yet performed prior to arrival in ED

■ If team consults additional services such as pediatric neurology, they are unavailable at this time but will evaluate patient if necessary

> **Critical actions**
> - Consideration should be given to additional seizure management including valproic acid, midazolam, pentobarbital or propofol drips
> - Stat EEG should be ordered
> - Blood work, cultures, urine and CXR should be ordered if not done already
> - LP should be performed if child felt to be stable
> - Empiric antibiotics should be given
> - Patient should be admitted to the ICU

9. STIMULI

None.

10. BIBLIOGRAPHY

Berg CD, Schumann H. An evidence-based approach to pediatric seizures in the emergency department. *Pediatr Emerg Med Pract* 2009; 6:1–22.

Hampers LC, Spina LA. Evaluation and management of pediatric febrile seizures in the emergency department. *Emerg Med Clin North Am* 2011; 29:83–93.

Nigro MA. Seizures and status epilepticus in children. In Tintinalli JE, Kelen GD, Stapczynski JS, eds. Emergency Medicine: A Comprehensive Study Guide, 6th edn. New York: McGraw-Hill, 2004, Ch. 125.

Rubin DH, Kornblau DH, Conway EE Jr., Caplen SM. Neurologic disorders. In Marx JA, Hockberger RS, Walls RM, eds. *Rosen's Emergency Medicine: Concepts and Clinical Practice*, 6th edn. Philadelphia, PA: Mosby-Elsevier, 2006, Ch. 173.

Neonatal cardiac arrest

Scott Goldberg and Yasuharu Okuda

1. SCENARIO OVERVIEW

A 6-day-old child is brought to ED with 2 days of increasing work of breathing, fussiness and poor feeding. He is full term from normal spontaneous vaginal delivery occurring at home. Today he rapidly deteriorated with cyanosis and respiratory distress.

2. TEACHING OBJECTIVES/DISCUSSION POINTS

Clinical and medical management

■ Identify and manage undifferentiated shock in the neonate
■ Appropriately identify and manage a ductal-dependent cardiac lesion
■ Consider the indications for and use of prostaglandin for cyanotic neonate in extremis

Communication and teamwork

■ Effectively communicate as a team during a complicated pediatric resuscitation
■ Develop rapport with parents and discuss patient care plan

3. SUPPLIES

Infant/neonatal airway supplies, IO device.

4. MOULAGE

None.

5. IMAGES AND LABS

■ XR30: neonatal CXR with cardiomegaly
■ Labs: ABG, CBC, BMP, LFT, clotting factors, lactate, urinalysis

6. ACTORS (CONFEDERATES) AND THEIR ROLES

▓ Nurse: generally helpful.

▓ Parent: concerned about child, not disruptive but may become so depending on play of case.

▓ Pediatric cardiology: if consulted early, they are busy and will be down shortly; if patient is arresting recommend prostaglandin. If consulted late will continue work-up on the floor.

▓ PICU: will accept patient to the unit but are otherwise indisposed.

7. CRITICAL ACTIONS

▓ Initiate appropriate identification and empiric management of the neonatal shock state

▓ Manage airway and use eventual ETT for airway compromise

▓ Use appropriate vascular access and fluid resuscitation

▓ Identify and treat a ductal-dependent heart lesion with prostaglandin

▓ Discuss patient care with a distraught parent

8. TIMELINE

Time 0

VS: BP 85/45, HR 180, RR 64, O_2 Sat 80% RA, 37.5°C, EKG – sinus tachycardia

▓ Summary of initial presentation: 6-day-old child arrives by private vehicle; child agitated, cyanotic, mottled extremities, obvious distress

▓ Unable to gain IV access, IO is able to be placed

▓ O_2 Sat will not improve with supplemental O_2

▓ PMH: full term, no prenatal care

▓ Surgical history: none

▓ Social history: lives with family

▓ Medication: none

▓ Allergies: NKDA

▓ Immunizations: none

▓ Physical exam
  ▶ General: agitated, weak, diaphoretic
  ▶ HEENT: sunken fontanelle, dry mucous membranes
  ▶ Neck: supple
  ▶ Chest: clear, tachypnea
  ▶ Heart: murmur of unclear location
  ▶ Abdomen: soft, non-tender, non-distended, umbilical stump clean
  ▶ Genitourinary: normal
  ▶ Extremities: cyanotic/mottled
  ▶ Skin: diaphoretic, cool, cyanotic
  ▶ Neuro: lethargic

▓ Point of care blood glucose 90

> **Critical actions**
> - Place patient on monitor
> - Check blood glucose
> - Initiate vascular access with IO device
> - Supplementary O_2
> - Differential of undifferentiated neonatal shock

Transition point 1: 2 minutes

VS: BP 60/30, HR 190, RR 40, O_2 Sat 75% supplementary O_2

- Increasing lethargy
- If fluid bolus through IO: BP improves slightly
- Broad-spectrum antibiotics should be administered
- Airway management should be considered
- Parent: wants to know what is going on, visibly distraught. "He was fine until yesterday! What happened?" Easily de-escalated
- If prostaglandin is administered prior to ETT, child will become apneic and O_2 Sat will fall (a common side effect of prostaglandin administration)

> **Critical actions**
> - Fluid resuscitation
> - Airway management (BVM or ETT)
> - Initiate empiric management of shock including antibiotics
> - Discuss care with parent

Transition point 2: 5 minutes

VS: BP 60/30, HR 100, RR agonal, O_2 Sat 70% supplementary O_2

- HR begins to slowly trend down to 30
- Patient should be intubated
- Prostaglandin should be administered
    - ▶ if prostaglandin administered: move to next transition
    - ▶ if prostaglandin is not administered: BP 00/00, HR 30, RR agonal, unable to obtain O%; patient will remain in this state despite any interventions until prostaglandin administered
- Labs: ABG, CBC, BMP, clotting factors, lactate, urinalysis
- Imaging: CXR
- Parent: still concerned with patient care/management; should be reappraised of patient condition

> **Critical actions**
> - Intubate patient
> - Administer prostaglandin
> - Review labs and imaging

Transition point 3: final actions

■ VS: BP 80/50, HR 170, RR (on ventilation), O_2 Sat 90% (on ventilation)
■ Patient is intubated, prostaglandin drip
■ Prostaglandin drip is initiated
■ Central venous access should be considered
■ Pediatric Cardiology: agrees with current management, will continue evaluation and management including echo in ED, suggest admission to PICU
■ PICU: will accept patient

Critical actions
● Continue prostaglandin
● Consider central venous access
● Post-intubation management including ABG
● Cardiology evaluation
● Appropriate disposition to the ICU

---

9. STIMULI

■ XR30: neonatal CXR with cardiomegaly

10. BIBLIOGRAPHY

Cepeda EE, Bedard M. Neonatal resuscitation and emergencies. In Tintinalli JE, Kelen GD, Stapczynski JS, eds. Emergency Medicine: A Comprehensive Study Guide, 6th edn. New York: McGraw-Hill, 2004, Ch. 13.

Colletti JE, Homme JL, Woodridge DP. Unsuspected neonatal killers in emergency medicine. *Emerg Med Clin North Am* 2004; 22:929–60.

Inaba AS. Cardiac disorders. In Marx JA, Hockberger RS, Walls RM, eds. Rosen's Emergency Medicine: Concepts and Clinical Practice, 6th edn. Philadelphia, PA: Mosby-Elsevier, 2006, Ch. 169.

Rohan AJ, Golombek SG. Hypoxia in the term newborn: Part 1 – cardiopulmonary physiology and assessment. *MCN Am J Matern Child Nurs* 2009; 34:106–12.

Steinhorn RH. Evaluation and management of the cyanotic neonate. *Clin Pediatr Emerg Med* 2008; 9:169–75.

Anaphylaxis in a patient boarding in the emergency department

Michael Falk

1. SCENARIO OVERVIEW

A 5-year-old boy has been sent as a "direct admit" to the hospital. The pediatric unit was full and admitting doctor sent the patient to ED for evaluation and admission. The boy was initially seen by his PMD for cellulitis and the PMD sent the child for admission because of the extensiveness of the infection. Patient had a "bug bite" on the right calf, which has become infected. Most of the boy's lower extremity is red, swollen and tender and he has streaks running above the knee on his upper leg.

You are the ED team and have just reached sign out at shift change when the nurse tells you about the patient. He has developed a rash with itching and is suddenly very short of breath and wheezing after getting a medication. She has tried to page the intern but has not had a response to the pages for about 5 minutes. She is asking you to evaluate the patient because the father is getting upset and was already angry that they have been forced to sit in the ED all night waiting for a bed.

2. TEACHING OBJECTIVES/DISCUSSION POINTS

Clinical and medical management

- Recognize and manage anaphylaxis in acute setting
- Recognize and manage difficult airway in pediatric patient
- Recognize and manage shock secondary to anaphylaxis

Communication and teamwork

- Get a history from and calm a difficult parent in an emergency situation
- Disclose and discuss a "medical error"/complication with family

3. SUPPLIES

- Pediatric mannequin
- Glidescope or other advanced airway tool for difficult airway
- Bags of fluids
- NRB

■ ETT and laryngoscope with appropriate blade
■ Suction catheters

4. MOULAGE

Right lower extremity cellulitis with streaks running above the knee; hives and urticarial rash on rest of body; angioedema.

5. IMAGES AND LABS

None.

6. ACTORS (CONFEDERATES) AND THEIR ROLES

■ Patient: mannequin.
■ Nurse: helpful and competent but she is "carrying" too many patients and is angry about the floor not calling back.
■ Intern: should be very hesitant and confused; this is the third day of internship and he/she is completely overwhelmed and clearly showing it!
■ Father: initially very angry and entitled; he has been waiting all night, not slept and is tired and frustrated, as one would be if boarding in the ED. It does not help that he is "connected" and has "friends on the Board," which he is happy to remind the team frequently. He will allow himself to calm down, in part because he sees how sick his son is, and his anger should shift to fear and anxiety after 2–3 minutes.

7. CRITICAL ACTIONS

■ Recognize and treat anaphylaxis
■ Anticipate and manage difficult airway
■ Recognize and treat shock due to anaphylaxis
■ Recognize and disclose medical error to family member
■ Calm and reassure potentially difficult parent

8. TIMELINE

Time 0

VS: BP 81/49, HR 120, RR 28, O_2 Sat 100% NRB, 38.7°C, EKG – sinus tachycardia

■ Summary of initial presentation: 5-year-old boy in respiratory distress, with wheezing, stridor, tachypnea and increased work of breathing; has an urticarial rash with swollen lips
■ Father: clearly angry and yelling; wants to know "What is going on?" "Why the hell have we been down in this hell hole all night?" and so on
■ Initial interventions: one IV line on right side with antibiotic (ceftriaxone) via that access; on a bedside pulse oximeter and will need to be put on cardiac/respiratory monitor with pulse oximeter and BP cuff
■ Team should place second IV line

■ Physical exam
  ▶ General: increased work of breathing, but no stridor at this time; can barely speak, 1–2 words
  ▶ HEENT: slight lip swelling and complaining of "itchy throat"
  ▶ Neck: normal
  ▶ Chest: bilateral wheeze with decreased bowel sounds on the right; tachypneic, increased work of breathing
  ▶ Heart: sinus tachycardia
  ▶ Abdomen: soft, non-tender, non-distended, with bowel sounds
  ▶ Skin: peripheral pulses palpable but weak and slight cool extremities; hives and rash all over body
  ▶ Extremities: right leg cellulitis
  ▶ Neuro: patient is sleepy but arousable, cannot answer well secondary to respiratory distress
■ Father: will become more disruptive if team fails to talk with him and engage
■ Nurse: very helpful but clearly angry at floor team and should make comments like "Where are they? I have paged repeatedly!"

Critical actions
- Initial assessment/examination
- CR and BP monitors
- Calm and talk with father
- Establish second IV access

Transition point 1: 2 minutes

VS: same as before

■ Patient's respiratory status should slowly get worse; he cannot speak and is unresponsive by end of this time frame
■ Nurse: should tell team that the patient got worse while he was getting the ceftriaxone and he has a history of penicillin allergy, "Why did they give it?"
■ Team should
  ▶ start first bolus of normal saline
  ▶ recognize and identify anaphylaxis
  ▶ give epinephrine at appropriate dose and concentration: 0.01 mg/kg of 1:1000 for SC or IM; 0.01 mg/kg of 1:10 000 if IV
■ Labs: none available
■ Imaging: none available
■ Father: should start to make shift from angry to scared/anxious by end of this time frame

---

Critical actions
- Start IV fluid
- Give epinephrine
- Identify cause of allergic reaction: ceftriaxone

Transition point 2: 4 minutes

VS: BP 73/45, HR 130s, RR 18, O_2 Sat 91%, 100% by NRB

■ Patient's breathing is deteriorating and team should recognize need for immediate airway
■ Should set up and anticipate a "difficult airway":
   ▶ RSI medications requested
   ▶ preoxygenate
   ▶ ETT size and one size smaller for narrow airway
   ▶ rescue device
■ Team will need to continue to treat anaphylaxis with signs of shock: give second bolus of normal saline at 20 mL/kg, diphenhydramine IV (1.25 mg/kg dose), steroids (should be given IV)
■ Labs: none available
■ Imaging: none available
■ Intern: arrives and is clearly overwhelmed and upset by everything; nurse and father are verbally angry with him/her

Critical actions
- Recognize difficult airway and need for RSI
- Treat shock/anaphylaxis
- Control difficult situation/family members

Transition point 5: 7 minutes

VS: BP 71/42, HR 130s, RR intubated, O_2 Sat 100% on ventilation

■ Patient is intubated but remains tachycardic and hypotensive
   ▶ nurse should tell team that cap refill is 4 seconds and patient has weak peripheral pulses
■ Treat shock with third bolus, pressors (epinephrine)
■ Intern: at this point, intern should mention that the night team chose to ignore possible penicillin allergy ("he had a rash with penicillin when he was 2 years old") and gave ceftriaxone
■ Father: should be very upset and angry forcing team leader, or another member, to identify that what they did was "OK" and why
■ Team: should discuss "medical error" with father and explain issues
■ Intern: should be *very* upset, saying things such as "I feel like I am responsible;" team should also talk with him/her about "medical errors" and so on

Critical actions
- Identify and treat refractory anaphylaxis
- Discuss "medical error" with family and intern

Transition point 4: final actions

VS: BP 87/56, HR 112, RR 12–16, O_2 Sat 100%

■ Patient should be stabilizing and responding to fluids and epinephrine; needs maintenance fluids and last of anaphylaxis treatment (i.e. histamine H_2 blocker)

■ Team leader should call ICU and sign out the patient, notifying PICU of the cause of the anaphylaxis and its treatment, and the "medical error" that was made
■ Talk with father one final time
■ Father: grateful and apologetic for early outbursts
■ Disposition: PICU

Critical actions
● Fluids and last medication
● Sign-out to PICU
● Last conversation with father

9. STIMULI

None.

10. BIBLIOGRAPHY

Lane RD, Bolte RG. Pediatric anaphylaxis. *Pediatr Emerg Care* 2007; 23:49–56.
Santillanes G, Gausche-Hill M. Pediatric airway management. *Emerg Med Clin North Am* 2008; 26:961–975.

Ondansetron and long QTc syndrome

Michael Falk, Viril Patel and Kirill Shishlov

1. SCENARIO OVERVIEW

EMS and the father bring in 10-month-old boy who has a 2-day history of vomiting and diarrhea. Child has not been tolerating oral fluids today, has had a low-grade fever and has been oliguric. The child has a normal birth/development history and no prior medical history other than congenital deafness. They saw their PMD shortly prior to arrival, who gave the child a medication unknown to the parent (oral ondansetron [Zofran]) and sent the child to the ED for further evaluation. Examination reveals a lethargic child who is actively vomiting, tachycardic and with dry mucous membranes. The father continues to ask the providers to "Do something" and give his child something for the vomiting. Once given ondansetron in the ED along with fluids, the patient becomes unresponsive and goes into cardiac arrest. The team needs to recognize torsades and give magnesium to obtain ROSC. It is later learned that the child has a family history of prolonged QT.

2. TEACHING OBJECTIVES/DISCUSSION POINTS

Clinical and medical management

- Management of hypovolemic shock due to dehydration
- Recognition of prolonged QT and medications that can potentially contribute
- Torsades treatment
- Overview of PALS

Communication and teamwork

- Importance of obtaining complete history from parents
- Communication with difficult family members/parents
- Clear communication with nursing

3. SUPPLIES

Pediatric simulator.

4. MOULAGE

Thick liquid that can represent non-bloody, non-bilious vomitus.

5. IMAGES AND LABS

None.

6. ACTORS (CONFEDERATES) AND THEIR ROLES

▓ Nurse: facilitate medications.
▓ Father: has poor English skills, is agitated and persists on asking for medication to be given.

7. CRITICAL ACTIONS

▓ Recognize the child is in cardiac arrest
▓ Initiate CPR
▓ Establish airway and IV/IO access
▓ Defibrillate
▓ Recognize torsades and give magnesium sulfate

8. TIMELINE

Time 0

VS: BP 83/45, HR 160, RR 24, O_2 Sat 100% RA, 99°F (rectal), EKG –sinus tachycardia

▓ Summary of initial presentation: 10-month-old term infant, normal spontaneous vaginal delivery but deaf from birth; otherwise no PMH. Infant has a 2-day history of multiple episodes of non-bloody and non-bilious vomiting, diffuse watery diarrhea over 10 times per day and inability to tolerate oral fluids. Child's older brother had similar symptoms several days ago but these have resolved spontaneously. Patient's immunizations are up to date; there is no recent travel and no previous history of antibiotic use. Child was just seen at the pediatrician's office, given "some medication" which helped with vomiting. Pediatrician felt that child needed IV hydration and sent him with his father to the ED
▓ Initial interventions: antiemetic given by PMD, "Starts with a Z"
▓ Physical exam
   ▶ General: well develop child, awake but lethargic
   ▶ HEENT: head is atraumatic/normocephalic. sunken eyes. dry mucous membranes; no oropharyngeal erythema or lesions; tympanic membranes normal
   ▶ Heart: sinus tachycardia, normal S1/S2, no m/r/g
   ▶ Chest: lungs CTAB, no accessory muscle use
   ▶ Abdominal: non-tender, non-distended, hyperactive bowel sounds
   ▶ Extremities: normal
   ▶ Genitourinary: normal
   ▶ Skin: poor skin turgor, capillary refill 6 seconds, no rash/lesions
▓ Father: very agitated and distressed by his child's condition. He provides history as stated above. If asked more questions about the cause of child's deafness, he does not know the exact cause, just that the doctors think it is congenital
▓ Nurse: if the team does not immediately ask to place child on the monitor, she can redirect the team

Critical actions
- Place on monitor
- Get history of presenting illness
- Head-to-toe examination
- Calm the father

Transition point 1: 2 minutes (as soon as vital signs taken and initial history obtained)

VS: unchanged

- Changes in physical exam:
  - ▶ child starts actively vomiting
  - ▶ vomitus is non-bloody, non-bilious
- If patient receives oral or IV ondansetron, he stops vomiting
- If the team asks for any other antiemetics, nurse says either that they have to come from the pharmacy or that they are unavailable due to a national shortage
- Labs: none available
- Imaging: EKG with sinus tachycardia and prolonged QT (only available if the team asks)
- Father: as soon as the child begins vomiting, the father becomes more upset and is asking for "that medicine that helped him earlier;" if his demands are not met and the child is not given ondansetron, he threatens legal actions. He is very persistent until the child is given ondansetron
- Nurse: helps with establishing IV access but unable to do so after several attempts, looks for the IO gun if asked by the team
- Additional points: the team should obtain IV/IO access, give fluid bolus, order labs and manage vomiting. The nurse can redirect the team if some of these things are not happening

Critical actions
- Establish IV/fluid bolus
- Treat vomiting

Transition point 2: 3 minutes (child becomes unresponsive, beginning of PALS)

VS: BP cannot obtain, HR pulseless, RR apneic, O_2 Sat 60% on RA, EKG – few seconds of torsades deteriorating into ventricular fibrillation

- Changes in physical exam/condition: child is suddenly unresponsive, apneic, pulseless, cyanotic
- Labs: none available
- Imaging: none available
- Father: hysterical when child is unresponsive but if there is a team member explaining things to him, he quietens down and does not interfere
- Additional points: team should recognize the obvious deterioration in patient's condition and initiate CPR/PALS; specific airway management is up to the team. If

the IV/IO access has not yet been established, the nurse can redirect the team. The team will advance to the next frame when they have started CPR, defibrillated the patient and established an airway and IV/IO access

Critical actions
- Begin CPR/PALS
- Establish airway
- Defibrillate patient

Transition point 3: 5–7 minutes (PALS)

VS: BP cannot obtain, HR pulseless, RR apneic, EKG – ventricular fibrillation

- Changes in physical exam/patient condition: child is still unresponsive, apneic, pulseless, cyanotic
- Labs: none available
- Imaging: none available
- Nurse: assist with giving PALS medications and cooperates fully
- After two rounds of CPR, epinephrine, defibrillation, if the QT prolongation causing torsades is not recognized then the nurse reminds the team about the FDA warning about ondansetron
- Additional points: child will remain pulseless and in ventricular fibrillation on the monitor until magnesium is given; once magnesium is given the child will regain pulses and a blood pressure

Critical actions
- Continue CPR/PALS
- Give magnesium

Transition point 4: final actions (ROSC)

VS: BP 78/42, HR 180, RR intubated, O_2 Sat 98% on 100% O_2 ventilator, EKG – sinus tachycardia with prolonged QT

- Changes in physical exam: child is unresponsive but has bounding pulses and is no longer cyanotic
- Labs: none available
- Imaging: none available
- Father: no longer angry but very concerned about what happened and on the verge of being tearful; once the situation is explained to him the father no longer interferes
- Nurse: helps set up child on ventilator and if the team does not call the PICU for final disposition gently reminds them to do so
- PICU attending clinician: gets story from group and ask them about any relevant history; if the team does not connect the congenital deafness to QT prolongation, then remind them about Jervell–Lange–Nilens syndrome, which causes congenital QT prolongation and deafness
- Disposition: PICU attending clinician accepts patient

Critical action
- Call PICU for proper disposition of patient

9. STIMULI

None.

10. BIBLIOGRAPHY

Chameides L, Samson RA, Schexnayder, MS, Hazinski MF. *Pediatric Advanced Life Support Provider Manual.* Washington, DC: American Heart Association, 2012.

Tranebjaerg L, Samson RA, Green GE. Jervell and Lange–Nielsen syndrome. In Pagon RA, Bird TD, Dolan CR et al. eds. *GeneReviews.* Seattle, WA: University of Washington, Seattle, 2012.

Pediatric death debrief

Christopher G. Strother

1. SCENARIO OVERVIEW

This scenario involves a futile resuscitation. The team must deal with difficult staff, call the end to resuscitation and then debrief and regather a distraught team for an incoming major trauma.

2. TEACHING OBJECTIVES/DISCUSSION POINTS

Clinical and medical management

▓ Recognition of a futile resuscitation and when to stop

Communication and teamwork

▓ Management of distraught team members
▓ Resource management skills
▓ Team communication
▓ Ad hoc debriefing skills

3. SUPPLIES

Moulaged child simulator or infant simulator.

4. MOULAGE

Multiple traumatic injuries/bruising on the mannequin.

5. IMAGES AND LABS

None.

6. ACTORS (CONFEDERATES) AND THEIR ROLES

▓ Patient: mannequin.
▓ Nurse 1: a new nurse that breaks down during initial resuscitation, crying, can't handle the stress/grief from the dead child.

■ Nurse 2: stoic, not helpful, angry, will not help the other nurse; barks at the other nurse to "get it together" and so on.

■ Chaplain/administrator: directs team to debrief/talk about the situation. Can prompt the team that the second round of patients "will be here any minute."

7. CRITICAL ACTIONS

■ Recognize futile resuscitation and the need to set team for incoming patients
■ Maintain good team communication and resource management
■ Manage difficult staff professionally
■ Debrief team after stopping initial resuscitation and preparing for incoming patients

8. TIMELINE

Time 0 (unveiling and case onset, in the middle of active resuscitation)

VS: BP 0, HR 0 (compressions), RR 0 BVM, O_2 Sat 80% RA, 35°C, EKG – asystole

■ Summary of initial presentation: team asked to step to bedside and told they are resuscitating a 2-year-old child who was brought in asystolic by rescue team after being found outside a car in a multicar accident. Team is currently 20 minutes into resuscitation with multiple rounds of medication, blood, CPR, intubation all done with no response. Child's mother (driver and a nurse in the department) is being resuscitated elsewhere. The team should be instructed to have one team member doing compressions and another bagging

■ Initial interventions: IV lines placed by EMS, prehospital 12-lead, etc.
  ▶ patient already has two IV/IO accesses, is intubated, on monitors
  ▶ patient has bilateral chest tubes placed

■ Physical exam
  ▶ General: unconscious, limp
  ▶ HEENT: pupils fixed dilated
  ▶ Neck: within normal limits
  ▶ Chest: CTA with BVM, no spontaneous respirations
  ▶ Heart: no heart sounds
  ▶ Abdomen: distended, ecchymotic
  ▶ Skin: cold, multiple bruises
  ▶ Neuro: GCS 3

■ Nurse 1: new nurse, seems stressed, distracted, having difficulty being helpful
■ Nurse 2: stoic, frustrated with Nurse 1

Critical actions
- Continue resuscitation
- Begin to consider futility
- Manage arguing nurses

Transition point 1: 2 minutes (chaos ensues)

VS: unchanging

■ Changes in physical exam: none
■ Patient will not improve with any resuscitation
■ Labs: none available
■ Imaging: none available; if asked, radiography shows multisystem major trauma (hemothorax/pneumothorax, fractures, pulmonary contusion, leg fractures, positive FAST etc.)
■ Nurse 1: a new nurse who breaks down once child is recognized by Nurse 2; crying, cannot handle the stress/grief from the dead child
■ Nurse 2: recognizes child as coworker's child and states "Oh s**t, that's Cindy's boy! And her husband is overseas." Stoic, not helpful, angry but basically will not say anything and will not help the other nurse, barking things such as, "get it together"
■ Chaplain/administrator: quiet at first but will eventually direct team to debrief/talk about the situation; can prompt the team that the second round of patients "will be here any minute"
■ The team should continue resuscitation and just as they are about to call the code, Nurse 2 will recognize the child as a coworker's child and husband is deployed overseas. She confirms the name and then Nurse 1 is overcome with grief. Both nurses require attention

Critical actions
- Recognition of futile resuscitation
- Manage distraught/arguing nurses

Transition point 2: 5 minutes (pronouncement/team decompensates)

VS: unchanging

■ Changes in physical exam/condition: none
■ Labs: none available
■ Imaging: none available
■ Nurses: both threaten to quit and go home as they cannot handle it any more. Get completely discouraged when they hear more trauma patients are coming in. Nurse 1 gets more and more crying/distressed; Nurse 2 gets more and more angry and argumentative
■ Additional points: as scenario unfolds at 3–4 minutes, an overhead page announces that there is a multivehicle crash with six occupants, two dead at scene and they are bringing in two adults and two children. The nurses state that they want to quit

Critical actions
- Team communication
- Management of upset team members
- Beginning of preparation for next patients

Transition point 3–6 minutes (regrouping/debriefing team)

■ Child should have been pronounced dead by the team by now
■ Nurses: will have completely decompensated and need to be gathered in by team leader and encouraged, debriefed and reorganized for the next patients; will allow consoling by team and listen to team leader/debriefer
■ Chaplain/administrator: quiet at first but will eventually direct team to debrief/talk about the situation; can prompt the team that the second round of patients "will be here any minute" and "I think we should all discuss this together"
■ Additional points: this should be the key time in the case with a focus on the team's ability to regather and debrief what happened, plus needing to prepare for incoming patients

Critical action
• Team debriefing

Transition point 4: final actions

If not already done, the team leader should describe how he would debrief the case to their clinical team.

9. STIMULI

None.

10. BIBLIOGRAPHY

American Heart Association and American Academy of Pediatrics. 2005 American Heart Association (AHA) guidelines for cardiopulmonary resuscitation (CPR) and emergency cardiovascular care (ECC) of pediatric and neonatal patients: pediatric basic life support. *Pediatrics* 2006; 117: e989–1004.

Cole E, Crichton N. The culture of a trauma team in relation to human factors. *J Clin Nurs* 2006; 15:1257–66.

Hunziker S, Johansson AC, Tschan F, et al. Teamwork and leadership in cardiopulmonary resuscitation. *J Am Coll Cardiol* 2011; 57:2381–8.

Norris EM, Lockey AS. Human factors in resuscitation teaching. *Resuscitation* 2012; 83:423–7.

Wampler DA, Collett L, Manifold CA, Velasquez C, McMullan JT. Cardiac arrest survival is rare without prehospital return of spontaneous circulation. *Prehosp Emerg Care* 2012; 16:451–5.

Infant abuse and the angry team member

Michael Falk

1. SCENARIO OVERVIEW

A 10-month-old infant is brought in by his mother because "he's not acting right." He has had 2 days of symptoms of an upper respiratory tract infection (URI) and fevers, but since last night he has been sleeping more, not eating well and has no wet diapers for over 6 hours. The father cares for the patient at night while mother is at work and he works days. When the mother got home today she found the baby acting this way. She has given acetaminophen and tried to get the baby to eat and eventually came to ED. The patient is "lethargic" and responds very weakly to being examined and to painful stimulation by the team. The patient has tachycardia, delayed cap refill (3–4 seconds) and weak peripheral pulses. When the patient is rolled or if the back is examined, there are a bruises on the back and buttocks.

During the course of the examination, one of the nurses will be become increasingly "upset" because of the child's abuse. Initially she is aloof and not communicative with the mother. But when the father comes in and it becomes clear that he is the abuser, she should become increasingly more hostile to the father and eventually initiate an actual fight or verbal altercation with the father.

2. TEACHING OBJECTIVES/DISCUSSION POINTS

Clinical and medical management

- Recognition and differential for a pediatric patient who is "lethargic"
- Recognition of AMS secondary to head trauma associated with an abused infant
- Stabilization and management of unstable airway in an infant
- Evaluation and appropriate consultation for an abused child/infant

Communication and teamwork

- Managing and controlling an upset/angry team member
- Communicating with parents in the case of suspected infant/child abuse

3. SUPPLIES

- Infant simulator: infant should have "jumper pajamas," requiring team to remove them

■ Appropriate airway supplies and IV material for 10-month-old infant resuscitation
■ Clothes for parents "appropriately" for ED visit (i.e. normal street wear, nothing "stereotypical")

4. MOULAGE

Infant mannequin will need to have bruises moulaged on to the back and buttock area, which should be a varying "ages" and colors.

5. IMAGES AND LABS

XR15: pediatric abuse, rib fractures (intubated view)

CT7: pediatric subdural hemorrhage

6. ACTORS (CONFEDERATES) AND THEIR ROLES

■ Patient: mannequin.
■ Nurse: should be female and is initially very helpful and appropriate. As soon as it becomes apparent that this is an abused child/infant should be come "quieter" and more "agitated." Once it is clear it is the father, she should become openly hostile to him and eventually escalate to actually "yelling" at him because of his continued denials etc.
■ Consult: PICU and children/family services or social work are available by phone.
■ Mother: very upset and appropriate. When abuse is initially suspected she should be horrified and very concerned. If she is asked, the child is *not* walking yet and has tried to stand up a couple of times.
■ Father: should arrive at 3 minutes or so, after the abuse has been discovered. He should be quiet if asked and say that he has no clue how those bruises got there. If he is pushed he should come up with excuse like "He keeps falling when he tries to walk" (which can be used as a prompt for mother to say "I have never seen him walk!") and other excuses.

7. CRITICAL ACTIONS

■ Recognize and evaluate a "lethargic" infant/child
■ Manage airway in infant/child with suspected head injury
■ Recognize and evaluate suspect infant abuse
■ Control an angry and out of control team member
■ Communicate with parents in a case of suspected abuse

8. TIMELINE

Time 0

VS: BP 76/46, HR 178, RR 32, O_2 Sat 98% RA, 38.3°C, EKG – sinus tachycardia

■ Summary of initial presentation: 10-month-old infant who is "lethargic" and responds weakly when being assessed and to painful stimulation. Has history of 2 days of URI symptoms and mother came home from work to find the child like this

■ Initial interventions: place on CR monitor with continuous pulse oximetry and BP monitoring
  ▶ head-to-toe evaluation of infant with age-appropriate GCS scoring
  ▶ recognize and start PIV
■ Physical exam
  ▶ General: the infant is lying on stretcher in "onesy" and not crying; responds weakly to painful stimuli with withdrawal weak cry
  ▶ HEENT: PEERL, mild nasal congestion, tympanic membranes normal bilaterally
  ▶ Lungs: equal and no crackles, wheeze or ronchi, mild tachypnea
  ▶ Heart: tachycardia but no murmurs or S3/S4, cap refill of 4 seconds, weak pulses
  ▶ Abdomen: soft, non-tender, non-distended, no bowel sounds, no masses
  ▶ Extremities: no abnormalities noted
  ▶ Neuro: weak cry to pain (V3), withdraws to painful stimuli weakly (M4), opens eyes slowly to pain (E2), giving a GCS score of 9
  ▶ Skin: bruises on the back and buttocks (should be "new" in color)
■ Mother: very upset and forthcoming; gives history without any issues and is very helpful to team
■ Nurse: helpful and appropriate member of the team

Critical actions
• Disrobe infant
• Gather history from mother
• Establish access

Transition point 1: 2 minutes

VS: same as on arrival

■ No change at this time
■ Team should recognize and initiate IV bolus with 20 mL/k
  ▶ if this done, HR will improve and BP will also improve
  ▶ should require second bolus to normalize HR
■ Team should recognize the need for definitive airway in infant with head injury and GCS of 9 and should set up or RSI
■ Team should recognize and discuss with mother the bruises on the back and how they occurred
■ Labs: none available yet
■ Imaging: none available
■ Mother: very upset when the bruises are pointed out. She should not know how they got there and can mention that she works nights and her boyfriend/partner looks after the baby at nights while he works days
■ Nurse: should be upset about the bruises but not overly obtrusive at this time

Critical actions
• Recognize critically ill infant
• Bolus fluids
• Airway management

Transition point 3: 4 minutes

VS: BP 91/57, HR 156, RR 32, O_2 Sat 100% NRB

■ Team should initiate and establish definitive airway: RSI with appropriate medications for a 10-month-old infant
  ▶ consider atropine
  ▶ once airway established, should confirm position with two methods (one *must* be $ETCO_2$ detection) and should get CXR
■ BP has normalized with first bolus and team should administer second bolus at 10–20 mL/kg
  ▶ if the initial bolus is 10 mL/kg, BP and HR can improve but should not normalize
■ Father: should arrive after or during airway being established
■ Imaging: XR15 should be shown to team after airway established and they should recognize posterior rib fractures (if team misses this, can have radiology called over at operator's discretion)
■ Father: gives story that the baby was crying a lot last night and not feeding well. Says had fewer wet diapers and he was up all night with him because of crying and so on but gets vague when asked when he "stopped crying" or for more details. If questioned about bruising, gives excuse about child walking and falling
■ Mother: quiet while father is questioned but should speak up when he says the child is walking
■ Nurse: should become increasing hostile to father and when the mother confronts him about the walking, she should become very angry. She should verbally abusive to him ("How can you hurt a child" and says all the things that many of us would like to say but don't) and continues to be disruptive until calmed/restrained by team members

---

Critical actions
- Inquire about abuse
- Intubate
- Manage angry nurse
- Manage father

Transition point 4: final actions

VS: BP 94/61, HR 143, RR on ventilation, O_2 Sat 100% on 100% FiO_2

■ Team should:
  ▶ identify need for CT head and skeletal survey
  ▶ call either child/family services or hospital social worker
  ▶ call PICU attending clinician to give sign out; PICU attending clinician should ask them to consult ophthalmology for eye examination the next morning if they have not done this
■ Mother: visibly upset with father and not talking with him; can ask team what happens next
■ Nurse: has been calmed by the team members or is being calmed by them; should admit to having issues with cases like this and has seen "too many" of them

- Father: non-communicative but not causing any issues
- Disposition: admit to PICU

9. STIMULI

There are two main stimuli in this case: visual and imaging.

- Visual: the bruises on the back and the team *must* roll the patient to see these; if not the nurse can suggest that they do so. These types of bruise in an infant who is *not* walking or doing other activities are highly suggestive (some would argue that they pathognomonic) of child abuse.
- XR15: rib fractures; there is no way that a healthy infant can get rib fractures unless there is some major trauma and given this patient's history, the only reason would be abuse.
- CT7: if there is time, the team may be shown CT7 showing pediatric subdural hemorrhage.

10. BIBLIOGRAPHY

Preer G, Sorrentino D, Newton, AW. Child abuse pediatrics: prevention, evaluation, and treatment. *Curr Opin Pediatr* 2012; 24:266–73.

Squier W. The "shaken baby" syndrome: pathology and mechanisms. *Acta Neuropathol* 2011; 122:519–42.

Intoxicated father with child neglect

Yuemi An-Grogan and David Salzman

1. SCENARIO OVERVIEW

A 5-year-old child with unknown PMH brought in to the theme park's medical clinic after he was witnessed falling from a step while waiting in line to get on a ride. The child appears well but is crying; the child will ultimately turn out to have a possible fracture. The police were called to the scene because the child's father was intoxicated yelling at the staff. There are no other family members to be found. This situation deals with social issues, including dealing with an intoxicated father and child neglect. It is unclear where the child's mother is, if she is involved and whether or not the father has legal custody of child.

This scenario can be interpreted and manipulated to user's needs/discretion.

2. TEACHING OBJECTIVES/DISCUSSION POINTS

Clinical and medical management

- Management of intoxicated father
- Management of child with possible orthopedic injury

Communication and teamwork

- Potential involvement of child protective services/social services for possible child neglect
- Disposition and resource management for intoxicated parent and injured child

3. SUPPLIES

Child toy, bandages, possibly sling, empty alcohol bottle, street clothes, police uniform (extra).

4. MOULAGE

- Adult: disheveled (basically look like an alcoholic, clothes torn/untucked, holding paper bag with bottle, etc.)
- Child: tears on face, abrasions to right elbow/forearm

5. IMAGES AND LABS

■ XR16: child's elbow

6. ACTORS (CONFEDERATES) AND THEIR ROLES

■ Intoxicated father: stumbling, mildly combative, obstructionist.
■ Theme park staff member: to bring child in.
■ Patient: a 4- to 5-year-old child, either a mannequin or a real child if available.
■ Nurse.
■ Police officer (to bring father in): only if extra person/uniform available, otherwise not needed.
■ Physician at local ED: voice only.

7. CRITICAL ACTIONS

■ Immobilize the injured arm
■ Consult social work/child protective services
■ Initiate resource management with intoxicated father

8. TIMELINE

Time 0–2 minutes

VS on arrival: BP 90/46, HR 115, RR 12, O_2 Sat 97% RA afebrile, EKG – no monitor

■ Summary of initial presentation: 5-year-old child crying holding right elbow, brought in by park staff
■ Initial interventions: none
■ Physical exam
  ▶ Airway: intact
  ▶ Breathing: clear bilaterally
  ▶ Circulation: palpable distal pulses
  ▶ Disability: GCS 15
  ▶ HEENT: no head injury
  ▶ Heart: normal
  ▶ Chest: clear bilaterally
  ▶ Abdomen: normal
  ▶ Pelvis: normal
  ▶ Extremities: moving all extremities except right arm, cries louder when examined, superficial abrasions and minor ecchymosis and swelling to right forearm/elbow
  ▶ Back: no trauma
■ Theme park staff member: brings in child (potential scripting below)

Critical action
• Assessment of child's arm

Transition point 2: 5 minutes

- Father: brought in by either police or theme park attendant (not as a patient); is yelling at medical office staff, verbally combative, ignoring his child who is crying
- Labs: none available
- Imaging: none available
- Nurse: attending to child
- Police officer or park attendant: trying to control and redirect father

Potential scripting

Park attendant: "This child was waiting to get on a ride and somehow fell and tripped on a step. He didn't hit his head and I think he landed on his side. There was a drunk guy next to him who was yelling at everyone so police were called. I'm not sure if that was the dad or not."

> Team member (to child): Hi whats your name?
> Patient: Bobby (crying/whimpering)
> Team member: Do you have any pain?
> Patient: My arms hurts (points to elbow)
> Team member: Where is your mom or dad?
> Patient: No answer but crying louder

Father is then brought in

Police officer or park attendant: "Hi, this man states he's the father of that child. He appears to be intoxicated and we couldn't find any other family around. We just got another call nearby so we need to leave, but call us if you need us and we'll be back to check on him later."

> Father to child: Stop crying! You're being such a baby!

Critical actions
- Placement of sling/splint
- Ordering radiography

Transition point 5–6 minutes

VS: no change

- Changes in physical exam/patient condition: none
- Labs: none available
- Imaging: elbow radiography available
  - ▶ no obvious fracture on radiograph, but still crying in pain
  - ▶ bandage/sling/immobilization per team
- Additional points: none

Transition point: final actions 6–8 minutes

VS: no change

- Changes in physical exam: none
- Nurse 1: If team has not called social work then should prompt, "What should we do with this child? He can't go back with his drunk dad. Should we call social services?" "Also, should we transfer to ED" if team has not already

■ Disposition: team to call social work/child protective services and arrange transport to local ED

Critical actions
- Call social work department
- Arrange transport

9. *STIMULI*

■ XR16: child's elbow

10. BIBLIOGRAPHY

Berkowitz CD. Child abuse and neglect. In Tintinalli JE, Stapczynski JS, Cline DM et al. eds. *Tintinalli's Emergency Medicine: A Comprehensive Study Guide*, 7th edn. New York: McGraw-Hill, 2011, Ch. 290.

Horowitz JR. Pediatric orthopedic emergencies. In Adams JG ed. *Emergency Medicine Clinical Essentials*, 2nd edn. Philadelphia, PA: Elsevier-Saunders, 2012, Ch. 25.

SECTION 8

TOXICOLOGY

Body packer

Jessica Hernandez, Brandon J. Godbout and Michael Smith

1. SCENARIO OVERVIEW

A patient presents after having a seizure at the airport. The underlying cause is hypertensive emergency due to cocaine toxicity. The patient is a cocaine "body packer," meaning that he has ingested condoms filled with illicit drugs for transporting. The team must identify cocaine toxicity and manage the patient's overdose, agitation and seizures, and interact with the family member.

This is a hybrid simulation case that begins with an actor and switches to a mannequin when the patient becomes combative and seizes.

2. TEACHING OBJECTIVES/DISCUSSION POINTS

Clinical and medical management

- Perform ABCDE; obtain a full set of vital signs
- Initiate appropriate work-up for an altered patient, including bedside testing for blood sugar and EKG
- Identify that this patient is a body packer and manage accordingly
- Identify and manage hypertensive emergency from cocaine overdose

Communication and teamwork

- Communication with family member using a translator
- Communication with team members
- Communication with consultant

3. SUPPLIES

- 1 condom filled with a white substance (either baby powder or flour)
- NG tube
- Water in spray bottles to sprinkle on the mannequin for "sweat"
- Airway supplies: non-invasive and intubating supplies
- IV tubing and fluids
- Syringes marked with medications

4. MOULAGE

- Confederate playing patient should appear diaphoretic (create sweat with water from spray bottle)
- Mannequin with sweat moulage
- Condom filled with white substance should be tied and inserted into rectum of mannequin
- Confederate playing girlfriend should be visibly pregnant, (create a gravid-appearing abdomen using sheets or pillows)

5. IMAGES AND LABS

- EKG14: widened QRS
- XR3: normal male intubated CXR
- XR25 Abdomen with intestinal distention and outline of cocaine-filled condoms
- If requested, the following labs will be provided:
  - bedside blood sugar 80
  - CBC with mild leukocytosis
  - BMP with increased BUN/creatinine indicative of acute renal failure

6. ACTORS (CONFEDERATES) AND THEIR ROLES

- Patient: hybrid case with an actor playing the first part as the combative delirious patient but case switches to simulator when patient becomes unresponsive.
- Nurse: helpful, relegates all decision making to the team; if team does not realize that patient is a body packer, the nurse will bring attention to the condom found in the rectum.
- Pregnant girlfriend: mostly helpful and cooperative with team, but speaks only Spanish. She will reveal information about patient's illegal drug trafficking activities if team makes a concerted effort to communicate with her using a translator.
- Translator: helpful, serves to bridge communication between girlfriend and team.
- Consult toxicologist: mostly helpful, will give recommendations for management.

7. CRITICAL ACTIONS

- Perform ABCDE
- Initiate an altered mental status work-up, including bedside testing and broad work-up
- Identify that patient is a body packer and diagnose hypertensive emergency due to cocaine overdose
- Manage seizure with benzodiazepines
- Institute aggressive airway management
- Manage cocaine overdose/packet ingestion with consideration for bicarbonate administration, whole bowel irrigation, toxicology consult, possible surgical management

■ Start appropriate treatment of high BP in setting of cocaine overdose, avoiding unopposed adrenergic tone
■ Demonstrate appropriate communication skills with team members, girlfriend, translator and consulting physician

8. TIMELINE

Time 0

VS: HR 145 (sinus), BP 220/110, RR 30, 100.3°F, O_2 Sat 95% RA

■ Summary of initial presentation: man brought in by EMS on stretcher post-ictal, minimally responsive and attempting to get out of stretcher; EMT reports "this guy had a seizure in the airport and he has been altered and combative at times since we found him"
■ Initial interventions: assess responsiveness and ABCs; assist in preventing patient getting off of stretcher
■ Physical exam
  ▶ General: opens eyes spontaneously, agitated, hot, diaphoretic
  ▶ HEENT: pupils 6 mm (dilated), equal/reactive (limited during actor phase)
  ▶ Neck: supple, no meningeal signs
  ▶ Chest: CTA, normal
  ▶ Heart: normal S1S2, regular, tachycardic
  ▶ Abdomen: decreased bowel sounds, soft, non-tender, non-distended
  ▶ Skin: no bruising, ecchymosis, or signs of injury, hot
  ▶ Extremities: no injuries noted
  ▶ Neuro: non-focal grossly, eyes occasionally opened, mumbling confused speech (Spanish), flailing extremities awkwardly, not following commands; no rigidity
■ Girlfriend: in background at time 0

Critical actions
- Assess ABCs
- Obtain history (EMS)
- Perform physical examination
- Obtain IV access

Transition point 1: 1 minute

VS: HR 148 (sinus) BP 230/120, RR 35, 100.3°F, O_2 Sat 95% RA

■ Changes in physical exam: worsening agitation, confusion and combativeness
■ Labs: blood glucose 80 (bedside)
■ Imaging: if patient is placed on monitor it will show sinus tachycardia, ST depressions inferolaterally with widened QRS (130 milliseconds)
■ Girlfriend: asks what is going on, "I knew this was a bad idea!" (repeated in Spanish until translator used); only reports "swallowing of drugs" if asked what girlfriend means by the above statement

Critical actions
- Must restrain patient or sedate
- Obtain history from girlfriend (use translator)
- Obtain blood glucose level
- Place patient on monitor
- Obtain EKG
- Begin IV fluids and O_2

Transition point 2: 3 minutes (patient seizes)

VS: HR 150 (sinus), BP 250/130, RR 40, 100.5°C, O_2 Sat 99% on O_2

■ Changes in physical exam/condition: patient begins yelling and then suddenly develops tonic-clonic seizure (prior to any sedation attempts)

The actor exits and the mannequin is introduced
■ Patient has persistent seizure despite IV benzodiazepines and becomes increasingly hypopneic with repeat doses, necessitating emergent airway management and propofol or benzodiazepine drip
■ Imaging: XR3 (post-intubation CXR clear with ETT in position)
■ Girlfriend: becomes tearful and hysterical

Critical actions
- Must recognize deteriorating vitals and sympathomimetic toxidrome
- Give IV benzodiazepines for active seizure
- Must protect airway
- Request STAT labs
- Start propofol or benzodiazepine drip post-intubation
- Consult neurology for EEG monitoring

Transition point 4: 6 minutes (post-intubation management)

VS: HR 135 (sinus), BP 240/120, RR (vent), 100.5°F, O_2 Sat 100% (ventilated), EKG – widening QRS

■ Changes in physical exam/patient condition
  ▶ patient intubated and sedated
  ▶ EKG14: increasingly widened QRS (150 ms)
■ Labs:
  ▶ CBC with mild leukocytosis
  ▶ BMP with increased BUN/creatinine indicative of acute renal failure
■ Abdominal radiography shows condoms in small bowel, with distended loops
■ Sodium bicarbonate administration improves QRS widening
■ Toxicologist: recommends whole bowel irrigation with polyethylene glycol (NG tube)
■ Girlfriend: volunteers "It must be the drugs he ingested" (Spanish) if team does not solidify history of body-packing at this time

Critical actions
- Solidify history of body-packing and recognize cocaine overdose
- Obtain abdominal radiography
- Prompt treatment of widened QRS with sodium bicarbonate (1–2 mEq/kg)
- Initiate whole bowel irrigation
- Consult toxicology

Transition point 4: final actions (patient resuscitated adequately)

VS: HR 120 (sinus), BP 198/100, HR (ventilated), 100.5°F, O$_2$ Sat 100% (ventilated)

- Changes in physical exam: VS improving with correct treatment
- Initiate appropriate BP control
  - ▶ patient codes to pulseless ventricular tachycardia with beta-blocker administration
  - ▶ prompt defibrillation returns circulation and case resumes
- Surgical team: consulted and requests patient is expedited to operation room
- Discuss surgical management with girlfriend
- Disposition: to surgery

Critical actions
- Continue sodium bicarbonate until QRS normalization
- Initiate BP control (avoiding unopposed alpha effect medications)
- Consult surgery for operative management and removal of ruptured body-packing
- Discussion operative management with girlfriend (translator)
- Disposition to surgery

9. STIMULI

- EKG14: wide QRS
- XR3: normal male intubated CXR
- XR25: abdomen with intestinal distention and outline of cocaine-filled condoms

10. BIBLIOGRAPHY

Mandava N, Chang RS, Wang JH et al. Establishment of a definitive protocol for the diagnosis and management of body packers (drug mules). *Emerg Med J* 2011; 28:98–101.

McCarron MM, Wood JD. The cocaine "body packer" syndrome. Diagnosis and treatment. *JAMA* 1983; 250:1417–1420.

Multiple altered patients with carbon monoxide poisoning

Jessica Hernandez, Brandon J. Godbout and Michael Falk

1. SCENARIO OVERVIEW

Three days after an earthquake in the suburbs of northern California which took out power supplies, a family of two –a 36-year-old woman and a 6-month-old infant girl – is at home and is checked by the mother's sibling, who finds her unresponsive, calls 911 and EMS brings her to the hospital. Mother arrives in critical condition requiring active resuscitation. Child arrives later, altered but stable. The team must identify and manage carbon monoxide (CO) poisoning. The woman has been using a gasoline-powered backup generator to provide electricity. The information regarding the generator, which is the cause of the CO poisoning, will not initially be given to the team.

This is a multiple patient scenario requiring an adult and a pediatric simulator.

2. TEACHING OBJECTIVES/DISCUSSION POINTS

Clinical and medical management

- Effective management of multiple patients
- Perform ABCDE; obtain a full set of vital signs
- Initiate appropriate work-up for an altered patient, including bedside testing for blood sugar, EKG, ABG
- Identification of CO poisoning
- Treatment of CO toxicity

Communication and teamwork

- Effective communication with EMS, family and consultants

3. SUPPLIES

- Moulage make-up for infant
- Female clothing

4. MOULAGE

- Adult female mannequin with women's clothing
- Infant mannequin with diaper on and moulage make-up to create a "mottled" appearance of the skin

5. IMAGES AND LABS

Provided only upon specific request.

Mother
- EKG1: sinus tachycardia
- XR24: CXR with non-cardiogenic pulmonary edema
- CT11: head CT in carbon monoxide poisoning; symmetric low attenuation in cerebellum, globus pallidus and caudate nuclei
- Labs: toxicology screen, CBC, BUN/creatinine, cardiac markers, ABG
- CO-oximetry (nurse takes time to find CO-oximeter): 34%

Infant
- EKG8: sinus tachycardia, pediatric
- Mildly elevated BUN/creatinine
- XR4: normal infant CXR
- Labs: blood glucose, toxicology screen

6. ACTORS (CONFEDERATES) AND THEIR ROLES

- EMS: responsible for giving report to the team when patient (mother) is brought to hospital; generally helpful and not obstructive.
- Nurse: neither helpful nor obstructive; takes direction from the team.
- Sibling: brings infant patient to hospital and provides information regarding generator use; generally helpful.

7. CRITICAL ACTIONS

- Perform ABCDE
- Resuscitate and stabilize patients
- Initiate altered mental status work-up
- Identify carbon monoxide poisoning
- Treat carbon monoxide poisoning (high-flow O_2, hyperbaric chamber)
- Demonstrate appropriate communication and professional skills

8. TIMELINE

Time 0

Mother
VS: BP 90/60, HR 135, RR 22, O_2 Sat 96% NRB, 37.0°C, EKG – sinus tachycardia

- Summary of initial presentation: 33-year-old woman, found at home unresponsive, GCS 9 (eyes 2, motor 4, voice 3). Patient has history of depression. EMS comments that it was difficult to obtain history from family member at the scene, secondary to

the very loud background noise from the generator. However, the family member is on his/her way to the hospital (EMS unaware of infant patient left at home)
- ■ EMS: states that they just "scooped and ran;" comments on difficulty in obtaining a history secondary to loud background noise from generator
- ■ Physical exam
  - ▶ General: well-developed female
  - ▶ HEENT: atraumatic, pupils equal/reactive
  - ▶ Heart: tachycardic, regular, no murmurs
  - ▶ Chest: rales diffuse bilaterally
  - ▶ Abdomen: soft, non-tender
  - ▶ Skin: pale, cool
  - ▶ Neuro: GCS 9, no focal neurological deficits
- ■ Nurse: assists with resuscitation as directed by the team

---

Critical actions
- Assess ABCs
- Gain IV access
- Obtain history
- Perform physical examination
- Place patient on monitors

Transition point 1: 2 minutes

Mother
VS: BP 90/60, HR 140, RR 24, O_2 Sat 95% NRB

- ■ Changes in physical exam: none
- ■ If fluids are administered, BP will improve
- ■ If team obtains IV access and administers dextrose-50 then patient's blood glucose will improve but there will only be a mild improvement in mental status
- ■ If team decides to intubate, pulse oximetry will improve
- ■ Labs: blood glucose 66
- ■ Imaging available upon request: EKG1 showing sinus tachycardia
- ■ EMS: no longer present unless team requests them to stay
- ■ Nurse: assists the team as directed during resuscitation; comments, "Is this arterial blood? It is bright red" during blood draw if labs are requested

---

Critical actions
- Recognize low blood glucose and treat with dextrose-50
- Request laboratory studies
- Request and interpret EKG
- Request CXR, head CT
- Consider intubation
- IV fluid administration

Transition point 2: 4 minutes

Infant
Infant is brought in by mother's sibling who found the infant in the home in a far back room with a cracked open window. Sibling says there is no PMH; infant presents with lethargy.

VS: BP 72/54, HR 155, RR 30, O_2 Sat 97% RA, 37.4°C

■ Physical exam/condition
  ▶ General: well developed female infant
  ▶ HEENT: atraumatic, pupils equal/reactive, normal fontanels
  ▶ Heart: tachycardic, regular, no murmurs
  ▶ Chest: normal breath sounds
  ▶ Abdomen: soft,non-tender
  ▶ Skin: mottled
  ▶ Neuro: lethargic, moves all extremeties
■ If infant given O_2, her mental status will improve
■ If fluids are administered, her BP will increase
■ Labs: blood glucose 66
■ Sibling: *emphasizes* history of closed doors and having to break in via windows; repeatedly mentions the loud generator and smell of gasoline and states, "Not sure if she even knows how to use that thing"

Critical actions
• Assess ABCs
• Gain IV/IO access
• Place infant on monitors
• Communication with sibling
• Identify CO poisoning
• Obtain blood glucose

Transition point 3: 6 minutes

Infant
VS: stable

■ Labs: available only if specifically requested
  ▶ mildly elevated WBC
  ▶ mildly elevated BUN/creatinine, mildy elevated CPK
  ▶ normal toxicology screen
  ▶ blood glucose 65
  ▶ carboxyhemoglobin via CO-oximetry 18%
  ▶ ABG on O_2 pH 7.4, PCO_2 35, PO_2 120, O_2 Sat 98% (calculated, without CO-oximetry)
■ Imaging available only if specifically requested: XR4 (normal infant CXR)

Mother
VS:

■ ▶ if intubated, improvement of O_2 Sat and RR
  ▶ if not intubated patient decompensates
■ Labs: available only if specifically requested
  ▶ mildly elevated WBC
  ▶ prerenal failure with elevated BUN/creatinine, elevated CPK

▸ elevated troponin

▸ carboxyhemoglobin via CO-oximetry 34%

▸ normal toxicology screen otherwise

▸ ABG on O_2 pH 7.36, PCO_2 33, PO_2 153, O_2 Sat 99% (calculated without CO-oximetry)

■ Imaging available only if specifically requested

▸ XR24: CXR with non-cardiogenic pulmonary edema

▸ CT11: head CT in CO poisoning; symmetric low attenuation in cerebellum, globus pallidus and caudate nuclei

Nurse

If team does not recognize CO toxicity, nurse will state, "Can't you get carbon monoxide poisoning from a generator?"

Critical actions
• Administer 100% O_2 for CO toxicity
• Toxicology consult
• Consider for hyperbaric O_2 therapy

Transition point 4: final actions

■ If both patients are resuscitated adequately VSs will stabilize

■ Sibling: requests update

■ Disposition

▸ ICU for mother

▸ PICU for infant

▸ consideration for hyperbaric treatment

Critical actions
• Communicate with sibling regarding disposition
• Consider transfer to facility with hyperbaric chamber
• Consider disposition to ICU

9. STIMULI

■ EKG1: sinus tachycardia

■ XR24: CXR (adult) with non-cardiogenic pulmonary edema

■ XR4: normal infant CXR

■ CT11: head CT in carbon monoxide poisoning; symmetric low attenuation in cerebellum, globus pallidus and caudate nuclei

■ EKG8: pediatric sinus tachycardia

■ Mother's labs:

▸ normal toxicology screen

▸ WBC mildly elevated

▸ prerenal failure with elevated BUN/creatinine

▸ elevated CPK

▸ elevated troponin

- ▶ blood glucose 66
- ▶ carboxyhemoglobin via CO-oximetry (nurse takes time to find CO-oximeter): 34%
- ▶ ABG on O_2: pH 7.36, PCO_2 33, PO_2 153, O_2 Sat 97%
- ▪ Infant's labs
  - ▶ blood glucose 65
  - ▶ toxicology screen normal
  - ▶ mildly elevated WBC
  - ▶ mildly elevated BUN/creatinine, mildy elevated CPK
  - ▶ normal toxicology screen
  - ▶ carboxyhemoglobin via CO-oximetry 18%
  - ▶ ABG on O_2 pH 7.4, PCO_2 35, PO_2 120, O_2 Sat 98% (calculated, without CO-oximetry)

10. BIBLIOGRAPHY

Weaver LK, Hopkins RO, Chan KJ, et al. Hyperbaric oxygen for acute carbon monoxide poisoning. *N Engl J Med* 2002; 347:1057–67.

Weaver LK, Valentine KJ, Hopkins RO. Carbon monoxide poisoning: risk factors for cognitive sequelae and the role of hyperbaric oxygen. *Am J Respir Crit Care Med* 2007; 176:491–7.

HazMat/decontamination response with complicated communication

Jared M. Kutzin

1. SCENARIO OVERVIEW

The decontamination team/unit in ED has been activated by EMS for an incoming patient. EMS responded to an apartment for an "unknown medical emergency." Upon arrival, they found a 20-year-old man who is only responsive to pain. EMS immediately assessed and evacuated the patient from the scene and transported him to the hospital where he seemed more alert and more agitated. The patient's apartment had a small amount of furniture (couch, mattress, table, folding chairs and an old TV) and assorted chemicals. The police, fire department and hazardous materials unit were notified and a quick decontamination of the patient was done in the field. Due to the unknown source of exposure and the patient's critical condition, immediate transportation to the hospital was initiated with secondary decontamination upon arrival. The patient arrives in respiratory distress, responsive to voice, with tearing eyes and blistering necrotic ulcers on his skin and areas of erythema on his chest, neck and arms. At this point he is agitated and screaming in discomfort. During the encounter, the patient's cardiac and respiratory status quickly decompensates necessitating intubation.

During the case, the clinical providers are dressed in HazMat gear and have earpieces in their ears connected to two-way radios on their waists. Siren sounds and "scene" noise is played through the two-way radios. At times, important dispatch information that may be useful to the team is transmitted through the two-way radios. The two-way radios serve two purposes: the first is to create an additional challenge related to communication. The second is to provide information about the causative agent.

2. TEACHING OBJECTIVES/DISCUSSION POINTS

Clinical and medical management

- Identify the source of exposure as a vesicant
- Recognize that no immediate reversal agent is available
- Respond with appropriate supportive care interventions (bronchodilators, intubation)
- Modify the approach to treatment due to the donning of HazMat gear (ex. challenge with intubating and/or administering medications with HazMat gloves)

Communication and teamwork

- Identify the challenges associated with communication while wearing HazMat gear (facemask, suit, and gloves)
- Modify communication techniques due to the HazMat gear

3. SUPPLIES

- Code cart (stocked), defibrillator, intubation equipment
- Medications: furosemide, albuterol, bronchodilators, *N*-acetylcysteine
- Two-way radios with earpieces for team members
- Sirens and radio communication

4. MOULAGE

A simulator should be moulaged with skin blisters/irritants that appear erythematous (red) with areas of necrosis. If possible, the areas should blanch when touched. The patient complains that the blistered areas are pruritic (itch) with other areas that resemble urticaria (hives).

5. IMAGES AND LABS

None.

6. ACTORS (CONFEDERATES) AND THEIR ROLES

- Mannequin voice.

7. CRITICAL ACTIONS

- Recognize the exposure as a vesicant
- Remove all clothing from the patient
- Decontaminate the patient with water (if possible)
- Intubate the patient for airway protection

8. TIMELINE

Time 0 (team already in HAZMAT suits)

VS: BP 110/55, HR 120, RR 30, O_2 Sat 95% RA, 36.2°C, EKG – sinus tachycardia

- Summary of initial presentation: patient arrives via EMS (BLS) complaining of extreme pain on the exposed parts of his body (arms and chest). The patient is agitated, short of breath and has an accompanying cough and nausea. EMS started the patient on 15 L O_2 via a NRB. EMS provide a limited report to the hospital decontamination team: patient initially responsive to pain but after removal from the apartment and during transport the patient became more alert and more agitated. The apartment had limited furniture and chemicals were noted to be surrounding the patient. Additional patients are on scene and the EMS unit has been called back to the scene to assist

■ Initial interventions: IV access, three-lead EKG (showing sinus tachycardia), initial decontamination done on scene
■ Physical exam
  ▶ General: alert, agitated, in pain
  ▶ HEENT: erythema on areas of skin that blanches, necrotic blistering areas, pruritis and urticaria in areas; bronchospasm and angioedema
  ▶ Neck: normal
  ▶ Chest: rales, congestion, bilateral chest rise, coughing, tachypnea
  ▶ Skin: blanching of the skin, erythematous ring, local necrosis
  ▶ Heart: regular, tachycardia
  ▶ Abdomen: normal, nausea
  ▶ Extremities: arms with blisters, hives, erythematous patches, local necrosis; legs normal
  ▶ Neuro: normal sensory and motor; moving all extremities; alert, orientated to person/place/time
■ Siren: continually played through the two-way radio

Critical actions
- Don HazMat suits
- Remove patient's clothing
- Decontaminate patient
- Administer O_2

Transition point 1: 2 minutes

VS: BP 105/60, HR 135, RR 20, O_2 Sat 91% RA

■ Changes in physical exam:
  ▶ HEENT: cyanosis, tongue edema
  ▶ Chest: bronchospasm
  ▶ Abdomen: nausea and vomiting
■ Sirens and radio communication: over the siren sound a fire department notification is made reporting that the scene has been turned over to HazMat due to unknown chemicals on the scene

Critical actions
- Identify causative agent
- Administer bronchodilators
- Intubation

Transition point 2: 4 minutes

VS: BP 85/40, HR 140, RR 28, O_2 Sat 86% RA (if intubated previously, oxygenation should increase to 92%)

■ Changes in physical exam: cyanosis should improve if intubated previously
■ Sirens and radio communication: over the siren sounds, a HazMat reports identifying a tan-colored oil on scene

Critical actions
- Intubation (if not previously done)
- Medication for sedation to intubate (if available)

Transition point 3: 5 minutes (or sooner if needed)

VS: BP 0/0, HR 0, RR 0, O_2 Sat 86% RA (or if intubated previously 92%), EKG – change in rhythm to ventricular fibrillation

■ Changes in physical exam: unresponsive: cardiac arrest

Critical actions
- Identify change in patient's status
- Communicate to team members
- Begin CPR
- Remain in protective HazMat gear

Transition point 4: final actions

VS: BP 0/0, HR 0, RR 0, O_2 Sat 92% if intubated (lower if not intubated)

■ Changes in physical exam: unresponsive, cardiac arrest

9. STIMULI

Two-way radios with earphones are worn by each participant. Siren sounds are played continuously with intermittent reports from EMS, fire department and Haz-Mat sources reporting various information.

10. BIBLIOGRAPHY

Atkins KB, IJ Lodhi, LL Hurley and DB Hinshaw. *N*-Acetylcysteine and endothelial cell injury by sulfur mustard. *J Appl Toxicol* 2000; 20:S125–S128.

Centers for Disease Control and Prevention. *The Emergency Response Safety and Health Database. Sulfur Mustard: Blister Agent.* Atlanta, GA: Centers for Disease Control and Prevention, 2013 (http://www.cdc.gov/NIOSH/ershdb/EmergencyResponseCard_29750008.html, accessed 31 July 2014).

Migraines and beta-blocker overdose

Jennifer Johnson and Lisa Jacobson

1. SCENARIO OVERVIEW

A 45-year-old woman was brought in by her teenage daughter who found her napping on the couch, pale, and too weak to get up after failing to turn up for her daughter's soccer game. The daughter thinks the mother has medical history of headaches. The daughter becomes increasingly distraught and agitated when her mother does not improve. A social worker is available to assist the team if the team requests help from social services. Eventually the husband arrives with a bottle of Percocet (acetaminophen and oxycodone) that is not empty and a story of another medicine for headaches that he cannot find. The husband does not know what medications his wife takes, but he is able to tell the team that she has a history of migraines if the team asks him about her medical history.

2. TEACHING OBJECTIVES/DISCUSSION POINTS

Clinical and medical management

- Recognize presence or absence of toxidrome
- Manage beta-blocker overdose
- Assess for co-ingested substances and recognize acetaminophen (Tylenol) ingestion
- Demonstrate central line placement using Seldinger technique

Communication and teamwork

- Assign team roles
- Calm anxious teenager
- Enlist aid of other resources such as social worker, child life team or chaplain
- Obtain additional history from husband

3. SUPPLIES

Pacing pads, ETT, central line, empty pill bottle.

4. MOULAGE

None.

5. IMAGES AND LABS

■ EKG5: sinus bradycardia
■ XR2: normal female CXR

6. ACTORS (CONFEDERATES) AND THEIR ROLES

■ Nurse: is competent and can perform the tasks asked of him/her in an appropriate, timely manner.
■ Teenage daughter: arrives with the patient and frequently interrupts the team with her concerns about her mother; she questions their ability to provide appropriate care, is tearful and refuses to let go of her mother's hand.
■ Social worker: is able to calm the teenager and prevent her from further interrupting the team.
■ Husband: provides a near-empty bottle of Percocet, which suggests an intentional ingestion. He is also able to give the history that the wife has migraines but he does not know any of her other medications.

7. CRITICAL ACTIONS

■ Recognize and treat shock
  ▶ fluid bolus
  ▶ pressors (placement of central line)
■ Evaluate altered mental status
  ▶ trial of naloxone
  ▶ fingerstick glucose
■ Treat beta-blocker overdose
  ▶ glucagon bolus and infusion
  ▶ high-dose insulin infusion
■ Evaluate and recognize co-ingested substances
■ Enlist the aid of social worker or chaplain to console the daughter
■ Communicate with family members

8. TIMELINE

Time 0

VS only given after patient placed on monitor by the team: BP 80/50, HR 40, RR 14, O_2 Sat 98% RA, 98°F, EKG – sinus bradycardia

■ Summary of initial presentation: pale cool woman aged mid-forties on a stretcher; she is drowsy, will follow some commands but is not really speaking coherently, if at all
■ Initial interventions: patient arrives with no IV access; if team requests IV access, nurse is able to place IV line within 1 minute
■ When fingerstick glucose is requested, it will take approximately 1 minute to obtain a result
■ Physical exam

▶ General: drowsy, mumbles at best
▶ HEENT: normocephalic/atraumatic, pupils pinpoint
▶ Neck: supple
▶ Chest: CTA
▶ Heart: bradycardic
▶ Abdomen: soft, normal active bowel sounds
▶ Skin: cool, clammy
▶ Extremities: unremarkable
▶ Neuro: moves all extremities spontaneously, follows simple commands

Critical actions
- Put patient on monitor
- Obtain IV access
- Assign roles to team members

Transition point 1: 2 minutes

VS: BP 76/45, HR 40, RR 12, O_2 Sat 96% RA

- No change in mental status with naloxone
- No change in physical exam
- If patient is given a fluid bolus, then her BP will improve to 85/55; her pulse and mental status will not improve
- If patient is started on pressors, her BP will improve to 90/60, HR to 55
- If patient is given atropine, there will be no response
- If the patient is given glucagon, her vital signs will not change and she will vomit
- Labs: blood glucose 40
- Imaging:
  ▶ XR2: normal female CXR
  ▶ EKG5: sinus bradycardia, normal intervals
- In the first 2–3 minutes, patient will not have any response to interventions, including atropine, glucagon or naloxone administration

Critical actions
- Trial of naloxone
- Obtain fingerstick glucose
- Treatment of shock

Transition point 2: 4 minutes

VS: BP 60/40, HR 37, RR 10, O_2 Sat 91% RA

- Changes in physical exam/condition: increasingly altered
- Labs available (see Stimuli)
- Imaging: no additional imaging

■ From 3–5 minutes, patient will experience some improvement from interventions (if appropriate interventions administered), but VSs fall again before 5 minutes:
  ► minimal response to fluid bolus
  ► minimal response to glucose infusion (pulse 45, BP stable)
  ► no response atropine or calcium
  ► pressors: some improvement initially to pulse 55, BP 90/60 using epinephrine 1 microg/min and titrate
■ If GI decontamination is attempted, it can only be done if patient is intubated

Critical actions
- Toxicology work-up/evaluation of altered mental status
- Enlisting aid of social worker or chaplain to help with upset daughter
- Treat hypoglycemia, hypotension and bradycardia

Transition point 3: 5 minutes

VS: BP 70/50, HR 45, RR 10, O_2 Sat 91% RA, EKG – sinus bradycardia

■ Physical exam: no significant change
■ Labs: no new labs
■ Imaging: no new imaging
■ At the 5-minute time point, the husband arrives with an empty bottle of Percocet. "I found this on the couch. She takes some other medicine for headache prevention, but I couldn't find it"
■ If no appropriate interactions attempted, patient will experience PEA arrest. Patient will have ROSC if 1 mg epinephrine is given

Critical actions
- Glucagon bolus then infusion
- High-dose insulin infusion
- Cardiac pacing, if not started on high-dose insulin drip

Transition point 4: final actions

VS (if patient is on insulin drip and pressors): BP 95/60, HR 60, RR 14, O_2 Sat 96% RA or ventilator settings if intubated

■ Physical exam: no significant change
■ Initiation of *N*-acetylcysteine can be considered
■ Disposition to ICU
■ Toxicologist can suggest propranolol as the etiology if team is not getting it "sometimes neurologists treat migraines with propranolol"

Critical actions
- Consult toxcicolgy/poison center
- Disposition to ICU
- Discussing critical condition with daughter and husband

9. STIMULI

- XR2: normal female CXR
- EKG5: sinus bradycardia
- Labs: normal with low glucose

Fingerstick glucose	40
Venous blood gases	7.36/41/35/28
Sodium	140
Potassium	3.5
Chloride	109
Bicarbonate	24
BUN	12
Creatinine	0.9
Hgb	15
Hematocrit	39
Platelets	189
AST	19
ALT	17
ALP	162
Lactate (mmol/L	1.9
Aspirin	<1
Acetaminophen	50
Alcohol	<10
Urine drugs of abuse	Negative
Urinalysis	Negative

10. BIBLIOGRAPHY

Bailey B. Glucagon in beta-blocker and calcium channel blocker overdoses: a systematic review. *J Toxicol Clin Toxicol* 2003; 41:595–602.

Engebrestsen KM, Kaczmarek KM, Morgan J, Holger JS. High-dose insulin therapy in beta-blocker and calcium channel-blocer poisioning. *Clin Toxicol (Phila)* 2011; 49:277–83.

TRAUMA

Blast injury

Kristin McKee and Lisa Jacobson

1. SCENARIO OVERVIEW

A bomb exploded 2 hours ago in the Copley Subway Station injuring 15 people; most are taken to the level 1 trauma center, but given the number of victims, patients start appearing in this ED as well. The patient will be more concerned with his pain from shrapnel than his pulmonary contusion, which will cause hypoxia and respiratory failure, ultimately requiring intubation.

2. TEACHING OBJECTIVES/DISCUSSION POINTS

- Identify the four types of injury from a blast (primary, secondary, tertiary, quarternary)
- Identify important components to gather in history (type of explosive, distance from explosion, location)
- Recognize and treat air emboli
- Manage the ventilation of a patient with blast injuries to the lung

3. SUPPLIES

- Otoscope
- Chest tube
- CPAP (continuous positive airway pressure) mask
- Mannequin

4. MOULAGE

Patient with multiple abrasions on face and shards sticking to clothing.

5. IMAGES AND LABS

- XR28 male CXR, pulmonary contusion, hemothorax
- XR29 CXR of male in XR28 after intubation
- US1: normal FAST
- ABG with CO-oximetry

6. ACTORS (CONFEDERATES) AND THEIR ROLES

■ Patient: with abrasions and shrapnel; more concerned about pain than his respiratory failure from his pulmonary contusion.
■ Nurse: to deliver medications.
■ Extras as family of patient: sister, wife, mother and friend have been searching for their family member and are very concerned.

7. CRITICAL ACTIONS

■ Activate disaster plan
■ Determine location of patient when blast happened
■ Determine if there is a need to decontaminate
■ Manage pneumothorax
■ Perform ATLS
■ Institute wound care
■ Control pain

8. TIMELINE

Time 0

VS: BP 115/70, P115, RR 30, O₂ Sat 92% RA, EKG – sinus tachycardia

■ Summary of initial presentation: 22-year-old man with no PMH walks into triage with abrasions, keeps complaining that his ears are ringing from the blast and is speaking *loudly*. He stayed behind to help others but a few hours have passed and he would like to be checked out now. If asked, patient reports standing against the wall directly adjacent to the subway car that exploded as it entered the station. He just noted a few scrapes, nothing serious
■ Physical exam
  ▶ General: anxious male, mild distress, having trouble hearing, multiple abrasions on face and shards sticking to clothing
  ▶ HEENT: tympanic membranes perforated (if checked), multiple abrasions on face, PERRL
  ▶ Neck: normal
  ▶ Chest: wheezing, tachypneic
  ▶ Heart: tachycardic, regular rhythm
  ▶ Abdomen: soft, non-tender
  ▶ Skin: shards in extremities, bleeding under control
  ▶ Extremities: moving all extremities
  ▶ Neuro: moving all extremities, having difficulty hearing commands to follow them

Critical actions
• Primary survey
• Activate disaster plan

Transition point 1: 2 minutes

VS: BP 115/70, P115, RR 30, O_2 Sat 92% RA, EKG – sinus tachycardia

- Physical exam: no change
- Team are expected to address two pathways: trauma management (ABCDE) and the wheezing
  - place patient on O_2: minimal improvement in saturation
  - trial of nebulized bronchodilator: no improvement in wheezing
  - pain control: will improve tachycardia
  - wound care and tetanus
- Imaging:
  - FAST: normal (US1)
  - CXR: pulmonary contusion
- Patient: some of the shrapnel injuries will bother him and he will whine about the pain in leg/arm and ringing in his ears as a constant distractor from any focus on his breathing

Critical actions
- Recognize and treat respiratory distress
- Recognize and treat traumatic injuries

Transition point 2: 4 minutes

VS: BP 115/70, P115, RR 30, O_2 Sat 92% RA, EKG – sinus tachycardia

- Physical exam: persistent hypoxia, respiratory distress
  - team should initiate BiPAP, nebulized bronchodilator or intubation
- Labs:
  - ABG pH 7.38, PCO_2 30, PO_2 60
  - CO-oximetry 15
  - recognize the level of carboxyhemoglobin; the team may consider treating cyanide poisoning but this will not change the case progression
- Family: arrives after having checked multiple other hospitals and finally found their family member here; team must manage this distraction

Critical actions
- BiPAP/nebulized medications
- Educate and manage family

Transition point 3: 6 mintues

VS: BP 115/70, pulse 115, RR 30, O_2 Sat 92% RA, EKG – sinus tachycardia

- Physical exam: massive hemoptysis, inability to protect airway, hypoxia
  - intubation required if not already performed

■ Ventilator management: ARDSnet or asthma-like settings *or* patient will develop pnumothorax, which will require intervention or patient will code

Critical actions
• Ventilator management with lung injury

Transition point 4: final actions

■ Patient must be dispositioned to ICU
  ▶ ICU attending clinician will need full debrief of patient's injuries and what has been done for him
■ Mass casualty management
  ▶ activate disaster plan if not already
  ▶ discuss with EMS
  ▶ divide resources to triage other patients
  ▶ determine need to decontaminate

9. STIMULI

■ XR5 (CXR intubated with aspiration) or XR8 (CXR with pulmonary edema): good approximations of lung injury before pneumothorax or can consider more severe left-sided injuries with XR28 (CXR with left contusion/hemorrhage/pneumothorax) and XR29 (CXR with left contusion/hemorrhage/pneumothorax after intubation)
■ US1: normal FAST
■ ABG pH 7.38, PCO_2 30, PO_2 60
■ CO-oximetry 15

10. BIBLIOGRAPHY

Dudaryk R, Pretto EA, Jr. Resuscitation in a multiple casualty event. *Anesthesiol Clin* 2013; 31:85–106.
Wolf SJ, Bebarta VS, Bonnett CJ, Pons PT, Cantrill SV. Blast injuries. *Lancet* 2009; 374:405–15.
Yeh DD, Schecter WP. Primary blast injuries: an updated concise review. *World J Surg* 2012; 36:966–72.

Multivictim trauma

Yuemi An-Grogan and David Salzman

1. SCENARIO OVERVIEW

A 48-year-old man with no PMH is brought in by the paramedics after a motor vehicle collision. The patient was a passenger using a seatbelt and with a child in the back seat (who also presents as a patient). The child is a 6-year-old boy with no significant medical problems. The car was "T-boned" on the driver's side. The other car's victims were taken to another hospital. There was airbag deployment and severe damage to the car. Both patients were non-ambulatory at the scene and had to be extricated from the vehicle; both are brought in as trauma activations, boarded and collared. The adult will ultimately be in hemorrhagic shock from an open-book pelvic fracture, and the child will be in spinal/neurogenic shock. Both patients will require early intervention and fluid resuscitation. There will also be a third patient who comes into the ED as a "walking wounded." This patient will require the team to use appropriate triage techniques and medical stabilization.

2. TEACHING OBJECTIVES/DISCUSSION POINTS

Clinical and medical management

■ Differentiation of types of shock
■ Management of hemorrhagic shock
■ Management of spinal/neurogenic shock

Communication and teamwork

■ Proper utilization and allocation of resources
■ Appropriate triaging of patients
■ Cognitive bias

3. SUPPLIES

Adult and pediatric c-collars, adult and pediatric backboard, arm sling, pelvic binder (TPOD or similar), IO gun/kit.

4. MOULAGE

■ Adult: ecchymosis to face and superficial abrasions to face, + hematoma right occiput, + seatbelt sign on chest and abdomen
■ Child: ecchymosis and superficial abrasions to head and face and superficial abrasions to left side of body
■ Walking wounded adult: none

5. IMAGES AND LABS

■ **Adult**
  ▶ XR17: chest
  ▶ XR18: pelvis
  ▶ US1: normal FAST
  ▶ CT8: normal head CT
■ **Child**
  ▶ XR19: normal CXR
  ▶ XR20: normal pediatric pelvis
  ▶ XR21: normal pediatric c-spine
  ▶ CT9: pediatric head CT
  ▶ CT10: pediatric c-spine
■ **Walking wounded adult**
  ▶ XR22: forearm/wrist

6. ACTORS (CONFEDERATES) AND THEIR ROLES

■ Adult: voice.
■ Child: voice.
■ Walking wounded adult (firefighter): actor.
■ Nurses (two): to assist with traumas.
■ EMS: to bring in both adult and child.
■ Neurosurgery consult: voice.
■ Interventional radiology consult: voice.

7. CRITICAL ACTIONS

■ Fluid resuscitation
■ Pelvic binding
■ Consult IR/orthopedic consult
■ Consult neurosurgery/spine
■ Splint Colle's fracture

8. TIMELINE

Time 0

Adult
VS: BP 105/60, HR 108, RR 16, O_2 Sat 96% RA, 97.9°F, EKG – sinus tachycardia

■ Summary of initial presentation: 48-year-old man, multiple scalp and facial abrasions, facemask, groaning and asking about his son

- Initial interventions: IV lines placed by EMS, boarded and collared
- Physical exam
  - Airway: asking about his son, yelling and groaning (patent)
  - Breathing: spontaneous breaths and present breath sounds bilaterally, no pneumothorax
  - Circulation: palpable distal pulses
  - Disability: GCS 10 (eyes 3, voice 3, motor 4)
- Nurse: present to assist with medical management; no prompts needed at this time

Critical action
- Primary survey

Transition point 1: 2–3 minutes

Child
VS: BP 75/46, HR 70, RR 12, O_2 Sat 94% RA, 98.2°F, EKG – sinus rhythm

- Summary of initial presentation: 6-year-old male with facemask, superficial abrasions and ecchymosis to scalp, face and left side of body
- Initial interventions: boarded and collared, unable to obtain IV access
- Physical exam
  - Airway: moaning very little, repetitively asking "Where's Mommy?" and "ow" and "stop"
  - Breathing: spontaneous breaths present, bilaterally
  - Circulation: palpable distal pulses
  - Disability: GCS 9 (eyes 3, voice 3, motor 3), not following commands, whimpering
- Nurse: present to assist with medical management; no prompts

Adult (secondary survey)
- Physical exam
  - HEENT: superficial abrasions on head and face, no lacerations, small hematoma right occiput
  - Heart: normal, no tamponade
  - Chest: clear bilaterally
  - Abdomen: difficult to examine, soft, no focal tenderness, +diffuse tenderness, multiple abrasions across abdomen, +seatbelt sign on chest and abdomen
  - Pelvis: pain with palpation, unstable
  - Extremities: moving all extremities, but not really following all commands, following some
  - Back: no stepoffs, no lesions, rectal normal tone
- Labs: none available
- Imaging: FAST negative
- Additional points: none

Critical actions
- Place IO
- Primary survey of child
- Fluid resuscitation of adult

Transition point 2: 3–4 minutes

Child (secondary survey)
VS: unchanged

- Physical exam
  - ▶ HEENT: superficial abrasions on head and face, no lacerations
  - ▶ Heart: normal, no tamponade
  - ▶ Chest: clear bilaterally
  - ▶ Abdomen: soft, +seatbelt sign over lower abdomen
  - ▶ Pelvis: stable
  - ▶ Extremities: will only move right side, barely, but not following all commands so limited examination because crying and yelling
  - ▶ Back: no stepoffs, no lesions, rectal decreased tone (if performed)
- Labs: none available
- Imaging: FAST negative
- Nurse 1: unable to get IV access; prompts with "I can't get an IV, I've tried multiple times;" will require team to put in IO

Adult
VS: BP 90/45, HR118, RR 16, O_2 Sat 94% RA

- Changes in physical exam/condition: no change in GCS/mental status
  - ▶ team to reassess patient and re-evaluate ABCs
- Labs: none available
- Imaging: repeat FAST negative, portable radiography of pelvis and chest
- Additional points:
  - ▶ if IV fluid given, minimal to no change in VSs
  - ▶ if blood given, minimal to no change in VSs
  - ▶ team identifies pelvic fracture (if not sooner), asks for pelvic binder and potentially calls interventional radiology or sends patient to CT scan to rule out intra-abdominal bleed

---

Critical action
- Pelvic binder placement

Transition point 3: 4–6 minutes

Child (starts to decompensate)
VS: BP 65/48, HR 65, RR 16, O_2 Sat 92% RA, EKG – no change in rhythm

- Changes in physical exam/patient condition: GCS/mental status indicates more confused, less responsive but still moaning intermittently
- Labs: none available
- Imaging: repeat FAST negative
- Additional points
  - ▶ if IV fluid given, no change in BP
  - ▶ if pressors given, BP increases to 88/54

Transition point 4: 6–7 minutes

Walking wounded adult

VS on arrival: BP 140/85, HR 98, RR 12%, O$_2$ Sat 99% RA, 98.4°F, EKG – normal sinus rhythm

- Summary of initial presentation: firefighter on scene injured while extricating patients; he is holding his left forearm at 90 degrees supported by other arm. Did not hit head, no loss of consciousness, no headache or neck pain; only complaining of excruciating pain in wrist
- Initial interventions: none
- Physical exam
    - HEENT: normal
    - Heart: normal
    - Chest: clear bilaterally
    - Abdomen: normal
    - Pelvis: stable
    - Extremities: left arm held at 90 degree angle, tenderness to palpation over wrist with obvious bony deformity, no open lesions
    - Back: no stepoffs, normal
- Nurse: if team ignores the patient, prompts "This guy's arm looks really deformed"
- Additional points:
    - one team member to address this patient
    - Order radiograophy and pain control until able to see image and splint

Adult

VS: unchanged

- Pelvic binder
    - if placed and patient given blood transfusion: patient remains critical but stable at **BP 95/50, HR 110**
    - if *not placed*: **BP drops to 84/46, HR 120**

Child

VS: unchanged, but O$_2$ Sat start to decline to 89%

- If CT scan ordered: tests come back negative
    - team should reassess and, given negative CT scan and hypotension and bradycardia, consider neurogenic/spinal shock
- Team should consult neurosurgery
- Team should consider intubation or bagging

Transition point 5: 7–8 minutes, final actions

Adult

VS: unchanged depending on above

- Changes in physical exam: none
- Disposition: identification of open book fracture, embolization by interventional radiologist or orthopedic consult for surgical repair

Child
VS: BP 65/48, HR 65, RR 16, O_2 Sat 89% RA

■ Changes in physical exam: none
■ Disposition: identification of neurogenic shock, neurosurgery consult and admit to PICU

Walking wounded adult
VS: BP 140/85, HR 98, RR 12, O_2 Sat 99% RA

■ Changes in physical exam: none
■ Disposition: identification of Colles fracture on radiograph; splint the arm and send home

9. STIMULI

■ **Adult**
  ▶ XR17: chest
  ▶ XR18: pelvis
  ▶ US1: normal FAST
  ▶ CT8: normal head CT
■ **Child**
  ▶ XR19: normal CXR
  ▶ XR20: normal pediatric pelvis
  ▶ XR21: normal pediatric c-spine
  ▶ CT9: pediatric head CT
  ▶ CT10:pediatric c-spine
■ **Walking wounded adult**
  ▶ XR22: forearm/wrist

10. BIBLIOGRAPHY

Baron BJ, McSherry KJ, Larson, JL, Jr., Scalea TM. Spine and spinal cord trauma. In Tintinalli JE, Stapczynski JS, Cline DM et al. eds. *Tintinalli's Emergency Medicine: A Comprehensive Study Guide*, 7th edn. New York: McGraw-Hill, 2011, Ch. 255.

Brunett PH, Cameron PA. Trauma in adults. In Tintinalli JE, Stapczynski JS, Cline DM et al. eds. *Tintinalli's Emergency Medicine: A Comprehensive Study Guide*, 7th edn. New York: McGraw-Hill, 2011, Ch. 250.

Hauda WE. Trauma in children. In Tintinalli JE, Stapczynski JS, Cline DM et al. eds. *Tintinalli's Emergency Medicine: A Comprehensive Study Guide*, 7th edn. New York: McGraw-Hill, 2011, Ch. 251.

Lin M, Mahadevan SV. Spine trauma and spinal cord injury. In Adams JG ed. *Emergency Medicine Clinical Essentials*, 2nd edn. Philadelphia, PA: Elsevier-Saunders, 2012, Ch. 75.

Paterson LA. Pelvic fractures. In Adams JG ed. *Emergency Medicine Clinical Essentials*, 2nd edn. Philadelphia, PA: Elsevier-Saunders, 2012, Ch. 81.

Traumatic head bleed/trephination

Kevin Reed

1. SCENARIO OVERVIEW

A 45-year-old homeless man found "asleep" on sidewalk and brought by EMS; he is well known to local EMS crews and hospital staff and has had previous EMS runs for alcohol intoxication. Patient will be intoxicated and have signs of increased ICP with an intracranial hemorrhage (ICH) due to coagulopathy. The patient is being treated at a rural hospital ED without neurosurgical coverage. He will deteriorate and require a life-saving cranial trephination by the ED providers with neurosurgical guidance by phone consultation.

2. TEACHING OBJECTIVES/DISCUSSION POINTS

Most hospitals worldwide do not have 24/7 neurosurgical capabilities and even more severe shortages of neurosurgical services are expected in the future. For salvageable patients, who have been alert but are deteriorating because of a rapidly expanding intracranial hematoma, the outcome is universally poor if they must wait for transfer to a tertiary care institution for hematoma evacuation. The most recent studies demonstrate that ED cranial trephination performed by EM physicians can result in uniformly good outcomes without complications. Opportunities to perform an emergency trephination in the ER are limited and exposure largely a matter of chance. A simulation model for cranial trephination creates a learning opportunity for all EM residents or attending staff for this rare but life-saving procedure.

Clinical and medical management

- Understand management of patients who have been diagnosed with an epidural or subdural hematoma
- Recognize the clinical indications for performing an emergency department cranial trephination
- In a setting where immediate neurosurgical consultation is not available, understand that while not common practice an ED provider can perform ED cranial trephination
- Demonstrate the procedural steps needed for correct cranial trephination and placement of an extraventricular drain (EVD)

Communication and teamwork

- Work together to identify critically ill patient
- Manage resources available in best manner to ensure the best patient outcome
- Effectively discuss situation with consultants and be able to put recommendations into action

3. SUPPLIES

- Commercially available life-size (fake) human skull under cover on separate table for trephination procedure
- Small (plum or peach sized) balloons filled with red thickened dye or jello to simulate hematoma; can substitute small IV bags (100–250 mL) filled with red dye as well
- Duct-tape to secure balloons/IV bags to inner skull table (one each side, allows procedure to be performed twice)
- Chucks rolled up inside skull underneath the "hematoma" to help keep fluid under "pressure"
- EVD and cranial trephination kit (prepackaged from hospital supplies suggested)

4. MOULAGE

Make-up for petechiae/bruising on extremities, possible caput medusa on abdomen; wrinkled clothes, old dirty socks; alcohol to be splashed on clothes for mannequin.

5. IMAGES AND LABS

- EKG5: sinus bradycardia
- EKG12: sinus tachycardia
- XR1: normal male CXR
- XR3: normal male CXR, intubated
- CT12: large intracranial hemorrhage and midline shift
- FAST: no images, verbally negative if requested

6. ACTORS (CONFEDERATES) AND THEIR ROLES

- Patient: mannequin, skull under cover on separate table for trephination procedure.
- Nurse: experienced but frustrated late in busy overnight shift.
- Neurosurgery consult: angry at being woken up but will be very helpful and supportive to ED staff once gravity of situation explained by team.
- Distractor(s) (confederates): not required for case but if possible can be major distractor if wanted (e.g. well-known alcohol-dependent patient in bed next to patient asking for lunch box, blanket, swearing occasionally at staff). If extra confederates available, can also have security available and called in to assist with this situation.

7. CRITICAL ACTIONS

- Identify signs of ICP due to ICH
- Interpret head CT scan with midline shift
- Treat ICP with at least two interventions, should include premedication for RSI
- Check coagulation studies and manage appropriately
- Perform cranial trephination with neurosurgical guidance by phone

8. TIMELINE

Time 0

VS: BP 157/90, pulse 58, RR 20, O_2 Sat 97% RA, 36.9°C, EKG – not on cardiac monitor (team must ask for this)

- Summary of initial presentation: 45-year-old man, somnolent, intoxicated and smells of alcohol
- Initial interventions: no IV line placed by EMS, fingerstick glucose 110 by EMS
- Physical exam
  - Appearance: disheveled male superficial abrasions to forehead, arousable to noxious stimulus
  - HEENT: airway patent with gag, no intraoral trauma, PEERL
  - Chest: breath sounds equal bilaterally
  - Heart: regular bradycardia at 56, no m/r/g, pulses intact in all four limbs
  - Abdomen: soft non-tender, stigmata of liver disease
  - Skin: ecchymosis and abrasions to extremities, no obvious torso trauma; petechia if asked by team (moulaged)
  - Neuro: will not follow commands; initial GCS 10 (eyes 2, opens eyes in response to painful stimuli; voice 3, inappropriate words; motor 5, localizes pain)
- EMS team: give typical "he is just drunk" report plus "He does this all the time"
- Team: should include at least two of the following: medical students, residents or attending clinicians; should have an identified team leader who should assign roles to other members
- Nurse: experienced but frustrated as it is late in busy overnight shift, fixated on odor/disheveled state of patient, not extremely helpful initially
- Distractor (if wanted): alcohol-dependent patient in bed next to patient asking for lunch box, blanket, swearing occasionally at staff
- Neurosurgeon: on call

> **Critical actions**
> - Calculate GCS
> - Assess airway
> - Identify bradycardia
> - Team leader assign roles to team members

Transition point 1: 2 minutes

VS: BP 206/100, HR 52, RR 26, O_2 Sat 89% RA

- Changes in physical exam
  - HEENT: diminished gag reflex; pupils now fixed and dilated on left (changed on mannequin)

▶ Chest: beginning Cheyne–Stokes respirations

▶ Neuro: rapidly decreasing GCS 4 (eyes 1, does not open eyes in response to painful stimuli; voice 1, no verbal response; motor 2, extension of extremities to painful stimuli)

■ If signs of patient deterioration not identified by team, then patient will have progressing hypoxia

■ Labs: none available but should be ordered

■ Imaging: none available but CT head should be ordered

■ EKG: sinus tachycardia (EKG12)

■ Nurse: facilitates examination by noting the funny movement of his arm when she placed IV line or bumped into him and noting belly breathing; can prompt team if not seeing change in VSs, "He does not normally do this" or "He looks bad all of a sudden… is he having a seizure" when patient postures

■ Team should identify signs of patient deterioration, order appropriate IV access, O₂, monitor, labs and CT head

▶ Labs recommended: CBC, CHEM 7, liver panel, INR/PT/PTT

■ Distractor: intervenes, occasionally swearing at staff, "Where the hell's my sandwich?"

Critical actions
- Establish IV access
- Identify signs of ICP
- Voice concern for possible ICH
- Order appropriate labs, CT

Transition point 2: 3 minutes

VS: BP 220/118, HR 50, RR 28, O₂ Sat 82% RA (95% if NRB placed)

■ Changes in physical exam/condition
▶ HEENT: loses gag reflex
▶ Chest: Cheyne–Stokes respirations, periods of apnea
▶ Neuro: GCS 3 (no response)

■ If patient sent to CT scan without securing airway first, he will have cardiopulmonary arrest on CT scan table

■ Labs: normal Chem 7, other labs pending

■ Nurse: assists with medications, asks if team wants anyone called for assistance (radiography)

■ Distractor: attempts to get off stretcher, needs forceful assistance to get back in bed

■ Team should:
▶ secure airway and recognize signs of ICP, otherwise patient will go into asystolic arrest
▶ institute RSI with lidocaine (or alternative), etomidate, succinylcholine
▶ order post-intubation CXR, NG/orogastric tube, Foley

Critical actions
- Secure airway
- Premedication for increased ICP for intubation
- Order CT head
- Order post-intubation CXR, Foley, NG/orogastric tube, check ventilator settings

Transition point 3: 4–5 minutes

VS: BP 230/128, HR 50, RR on ventilator, O$_2$ Sat 98% on 100% O$_2$

- ▣ Changes in physical exam/condition
  - ▶ HEENT: intubated
  - ▶ Chest: not breathing above ventilation, equal breath sounds
  - ▶ Neuro: GCS 3 (no response)
- ▣ Labs:
  - ▶ hematocrit 28, platelets 75
  - ▶ LFTs: AST, 220, ALT 300, ALP 360, total bilirubin 6 mg/dL, direct bilirubin 1.8 mg/dL, albumin 2.4 g/dL
  - ▶ INR 3.6
- ▣ Imaging:
  - ▶ CT head: large ICH with significant midline shift
- ▣ Nurse: assists with care of patient and medication/blood product administration if ordered
- ▣ Team should:
  - ▶ check post-intubation CXR, ETT position
  - ▶ recognize liver failure
  - ▶ order blood products to reverse coagulopathy
  - ▶ initiate increased ICP management in setting of ICH: elevation of head of bed, mannitol or hypertonic saline, sedation (propofol/alternative), MAP control or systolic BP <140
  - ▶ treat mild hyperventilation
- ▣ Distractor: intoxicated patient tries to get out of bed, spills urinal on floor
- ▣ Additional points
  - ▶ team may use electronic device/app/computer, consult pharmacy to confirm appropriate dosing of medications
  - ▶ Neurosurgical consultation to nearest facility available by phone

Critical actions
- Recognize ICH with shift on CT head
- Aggressive ICP management
- Order agents/blood products for reversal of coagulopathy
- Consult neurosurgery

Transition point 4: final actions

VS: BP 248/140, HR 42, RR on ventilator, O$_2$ Sat 93% on 100% O$_2$

- ▣ Changes in physical exam/condition
  - ▶ HEENT: intubated
  - ▶ Chest: not breathing above vent, equal breath sounds
  - ▶ Neuro: GCS 3 (no response)
  - ▶ Continued BP rise and HR decrease: now HR in 40s, still sinus bradycardia despite aggressive ICP management post-intubation
- ▣ Nurse: assists with care of patient and medication/blood product administration if ordered

■ Neurosurgery consult: lengthy transport time so recommends ED performed trephination and EVD placement; assurea team that they will be talked through step-by-step by phone

  ► if team refuses to attempt trephination, patient codes and is unable to be resuscitated

■ Disposition

  ► VSs improve to HR 70s, BP 140/80

  ► reconsult neurosurgical team at transfer facility to update status

  ► Medevac team should arrive in 15 minutes

Critical actions
- Recognize progressing herniation due to ICH
- Perform ED trephination and EVD with neurosurgical guidance
- Reconsult after procedure

---

9. STIMULI

■ EKG5: sinus bradycardia

■ EKG12: sinus tachycardia

■ XR1: normal male CXR

■ XR3: normal male CXR, intubated

■ CT12: large intracranial hemorrhage and midline shift

10. BIBLIOGRAPHY

Donovan DJ et al. Cranial burr holes and emergency craniotomy: review of indications and technique. *Mil Med* 2006; 171:12–19.

Poon WS, Li AK. Comparison of management outcome of primary and secondary referred patients with traumatic extradural hematoma in a neurosurgical unit. *Injury* 1991; 22:323–5.

Smith SW et al. Emergency department skull trephination for epidural hematoma in patients who are awake but deteriorate rapidly. *J Emerg Med* 2010; 39:377–83.

World Health Organization. Cranial burr hole. In *Surgical Care at the District Hospital, Part 6: Traumatology and Orthopaedics*. Geneva: World Health Organization, 2003, Ch. 17 (http://www.who.int/surgery/publications/en/SCDH.pdf, accessed 31 July, 2014).

Trapped in the elevator

Jared M. Kutzin

1. SCENARIO OVERVIEW

A maintenance man working on a hospital elevator neglected to place an out-of-service sign on the elevator. During final maintenance testing, the elevator is accidentally used by a 37-year-old male hospital visitor and a staff member. The elevator suddenly rises as the man is crossing the elevator threshold. The man's leg is amputated below the knee and the elevator is trapped between floors. The patient's torso is in the elevator while his leg remains dangling over the edge. The team arrives to find the elevator trapped between floors, with only 45 cm (18 inches) of room at the top of the elevator shaft available to communicate with and treat the patient. Inside the elevator is an emergency room patient care assistant (PCA) who is also an emergency medical technician (EMT-B). Because of the accident, the power has been turned off and the team is working with emergency lighting. Maintenance is notified and is coming to stabilize the elevator. The fire department, if notified, is 15 minutes away.

2. TEACHING OBJECTIVES/DISCUSSION POINTS

Clinical and medical management

- Recognize the importance of scene safety before attempting to treat a patient
- Assist the patient care technician in the elevator to complete an assessment of the patient's ABCs
- Demonstrate appropriate management of an amputated limb (bleeding control)
- Identify the need for additional resources (fire department/rescue services)

Communication and teamwork

- Demonstrate clear role designation
- Identify a team leader responsible for scene coordination
- Identify the importance of communicating with the patient care assistant inside the elevator and providing clear instructions to him or her

3. SUPPLIES

Medical response bag with cervical collar, backboard, stretcher, 4 × 4 gauze, abdominal pad gauze, IV fluids, IV catheters, patient monitor (cardiac rhythm, BP, oximeter).

Fig. 45.1 Layout
for the elevator
accident.

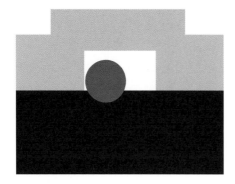

4. MOULAGE

An elevator shaft needs to be created. This was completed by using pipe and drape and placing the mannequin on a raised platform with pipe and drape above, below and to the sides mannequin to create an elevator opening. In Fig. 45.1, the circle represents the patient's leg presenting towards the responding team. The area above represents pipe and drape and the rectangle below represents a raised stage area.

The mannequin should be placed on the raised platform, approximately 1.8 m (6 feet) from the ground. Pipe and drape should be placed so that draping comes down to approximately 2.3 m (7.5 feet) from the ground, resulting in an opening of about 45 cm (18 inches). The patient's amputated leg should be actively bleeding, uncontrolled with direct pressure, and the other leg has abrasions and torn clothing. The amputated extremity should bleed and "squirt" until appropriately managed.

5. IMAGES AND LABS

None.

6. ACTORS (CONFEDERATES) AND THEIR ROLES

- Patient care assistant (PCA): is in the elevator with the injured visitor and can assist the team but is emotionally distraught and must be calmed by the responding providers before being able to assist. The PCA only assists if given specific instructions by the responding team, otherwise she/he is hyperventilating, upset and wants to know when she/he will be able to get out.
- Elevator maintenance: will respond to team's request for safety information.
- Extra confederates: behave as visitors and employees of hospital who stroll by to capture pictures of the "disaster."

7. CRITICAL ACTIONS

- Identify the safety of the scene/make the scene safe
- Communicate with and calm down the PCA in the elevator
- Assess the injured patient with the assistance of the PCA
- Control bleeding via direct pressure and tourniquet
- Safely remove the patient from the elevator

8. TIMELINE

Time 0

VS: BP 110/50, HR 120, RR 28, O$_2$ Sat 95% RA, 38.7°C, EKG – sinus tachycardia

- Summary of initial presentation: 37-year-old man trapped in elevator caught between floors; patient has an amputated lower extremity and abrasions and torn clothing on the other extremity. The elevator is trapped approximately 6 feet off the ground
- Initial interventions: a PCA confederate is also in the elevator, but no interventions have been started before the team's arrival
- Physical exam
  - General: alert, agitated, in pain
  - HEENT: head bruised from the impact, but alert
  - Neck: normal
  - Chest: normal, clear to auscultation
  - Heart: regular, tachycardia
  - Abdomen: normal, soft
  - Skin: pale, diaphoretic
  - Extremities: arms normal; amputation of one leg, bruising and torn clothing on the other leg
  - Neuro: pain in exposed regions
- PCA: extremely emotional, screaming that they need help; initially uncooperative (until spoken to and given specific tasks by the team)

> **Critical actions**
> - Ensure scene safety (make sure power is off)
> - Call for additional help (fire department/rescue)
> - Assess the number of patients
> - Delegate roles

Transition point 1: 2 minutes

VS: BP 102/48, HR 130, RR 24, O$_2$ Sat 95% RA

- Changes in physical exam: bleeding not controlled with direct pressure
- Patient continues to scream in pain; pain is 10/10
- Labs: unavailable
- Imaging: unavailable
- PCA: continues to be emotionally upset and causing chaos until calmed by responders and given specific tasks; when a task is complete they report back to the team but if they are not given another task, they remain quiet for 30 seconds and then start asking when they will be rescued
- Elevator maintenance: if called by the team, will respond quickly and advise that the elevator is not yet safe but they are working on making the elevator safe; at minute 3 they will report back to the team that the elevator is now deemed "safe"

> **Critical actions**
> - Request spinal immobilization equipment if not present
> - Decide whether to treat in place or move patient
> - Bleeding control (direct pressure)
> - Communicate with PCA inside elevator

Transition point 2: 3 minutes

VS: BP 90/50, HR 135, RR 26, O$_2$ Sat 95% RA

- Changes in physical exam/condition:
  - ▶ bleeding continues until tourniquet is applied
  - ▶ patient becomes less responsive as blood loss continues
- PCA: continues as above
- Elevator maintenance: if not requested previously, will report to the scene at minute 3; if previously contacted, will report back to the scene at minute 3 and advise that the elevator has been made "safe," meaning that the elevator will *not* move
- Onlookers: gather around the scene, some using camera phones, necessitating crowd control

Critical actions
- IV fluid administration (two large-bore IV lines with isotonic crystalloid solution)
- Rapid trauma assessment
- Bleeding control (tourniquet)
- Communicate with PCA

Transition point 3: 5 minutes: final actions

VS: as above

- Changes in physical exam/patient condition:
  - ▶ continues to become less responsive
  - ▶ continues to bleed until tourniquet is applied
- PCA: same as above
- Disposition: await assistance from EMS/fire rescue while controlling bleeding

Critical actions
- Decide whether to leave patient in place and await fire department assistance or remove patient with appropriate spinal precautions
- Institute fluid resuscitation
- Consider use of clotting agent on amputated extremity

9. STIMULI

None.

10. BIBLIOGRAPHY

Beekley AC, Sebesta JA, Blackbourne LH et al. Preshospital tourniquet use in Operation Iraqi Freedom: effect on hemorrhage control and outcomes. *J Trauma* 2008; 64(Suppl): S28–S37.

Markenson D, Ferguson JD, Chameides L et al. Part 17: First aid: 2010 American Heart Association and American Red Cross Guidelines for First Aid. *Circulation* 2010; 122(Suppl 3):S934–S946.

Mass casualty incident: "I'm never riding rollercoasters again"

Kirill Shishlov and Michael Falk

1. SCENARIO OVERVIEW

The team is called to the scene of a rollercoaster disaster and are responsible for the patients in their area. At this time there are no EMS units available for transport and it is the team's job to triage and stabilize the patients as they arrive from the scene of the disaster. While the team is only four people, there are resources available in the crowd (a paramedic on holiday, another EMT and a couple of bystanders with basic first aid skills) and it is part of the team/team leader's responsibility in this scenario to identify possible supports to manage the scene. As patients are brought in to the staging area, the team needs to rapidly triage and decide how to allocate their attention and resources. There are several "green" patients who require nothing more than reassurance and will act as distractors. Similarly, two "yellow" patients require no immediate medical care but close monitoring. There are two "red" critical care patients who need immediate resuscitation and will be the focus of the medical aspect of the case. Finally, there are two "black" patients whose further resuscitation is futile. The patients come in two or three at a time by EMS from the scene as well as walking wounded. The case will finish when both of the "red" patients are resuscitated and the hospital transport EMS arrives.

2. TEACHING OBJECTIVES/DISCUSSION POINTS

Clinical and medical management

- Initial stabilization and resuscitation of critically ill patients in mass casualty scenario
- Importance of a complete secondary survey and reassessment after the patient has been stabilized
- Immediate tourniquet placement on exsanguinating extremity amputation/injury
- Immediate needle decompression of a tension pneumothorax

Communication and teamwork

- Importance of triage during a mass casualty event
- Importance of allocation of limited resources

- Delegating different tasks to team members
- Ability to identify and utilize resources in a resource-poor environment, by using "bystanders" with medical knowledge

3. SUPPLIES

Airway equipment, IV setup/bags, intubation setup, IO kit, EMS monitor, bandages, CAT tourniquet, 2 EMS gurneys, 2 stretchers for the "black tags," EMS extremity splints, c-collar.

4. MOULAGE

- **Red 1** (adult mannequin): amputation of one of the extremities with bloody bandages and blood seeping through, simulated arterial bleed; minor other abrasions
- **Red 2** (adult mannequin): splinted left leg, including the femur; abrasions and bruising to chest wall
- **Black 1** (child mannequin): large abrasion on the head and bleeding from nose and one ear to indicate skull fracture; a small doll can be used
- **Black 2** (adult mannequin): large piece of metal moulaged through the middle of the chest

5. IMAGES AND LABS

None.

6. ACTORS (CONFEDERATES) AND THEIR ROLES

- Patients
  - **Yellow 1**: adult with minor head injury; abrasion on the head, slightly unsteady gait with mild confusion but otherwise stable and cooperative with exam/ directions
  - **Yellow 2**: adult with minor right shoulder injury and right arm splint suggestive of fracture; he is in pain, acting very entitled, demanding medication and to be seen immediately
  - **Red 1** (voice for the mannequin): slow lethargic answers, quietly moaning
  - **Red 2** (voice for the mannequin): has respiratory distress, speaking in short sentences; frequently complains of leg pain and chest pain
  - **Mother of Black 1**: young woman arrives carrying her child and is clearly distraught and hysterical. She is repeatedly asking the team to save her baby and why aren't they helping her. She can be calmed but needs to be told by team leader that her child is dead and there is nothing that can be done (in a gentle but formal manner).
- Paramedic on scene: will volunteer immediately even if team does not ask for help.
- Two other EMT, basic level: available but they do not identify themselves as providers immediately unless asked by team leader or members.
- EMS crew: bring patients but should *not* stay because they have to go back to the scene and help.

■ Green patients (confederates): several walking wounded who have minor scrapes/abrasions, walk in at different times, ask for help and are very cooperating when redirected.

7. CRITICAL ACTIONS

■ Complete secondary survey and c-collar placement for both **Red 1** and **Red 2**
■ Place tourniquet on amputation on **Red 1** and administer 1 L normal saline bolus (or 2 L if desired)
■ Recognize need for immediate access and use of IO on **Red 1**
■ Appropriately triaging patients at scene of mass casualty event and recognize medical futility with "black tagging" of patients
■ Recognize and inititate appropriate treatment of tension pneumothorax for **Red 2**

8. TIMELINE

Time 0

Black 1
VS: BP none, HR 0, RR 0, no O_2 monitor, EKG – waveform asystole

■ Summary of initial presentation: young hysterical woman holding her child who she says fell from roller-coaster, "very high," and she grabbed him and brought him here right away. Child hasn't been breathing since the fall, now about 10–15 minutes
■ Initial interventions: none
■ Physical exam
  ▶ HEENT: abrasion on forehead; blood at nostrils and ears
  ▶ General: no other gross deformities/signs of trauma
  ▶ Apneic
  ▶ Pulseless
  ▶ Neuro: GCS 3
■ Team leader or designated surrogate: should tell the woman that the child is dead and, if possible, designate an ancillary helper to console her
■ Goal is to bring in **Red 1** while the team is dealing with **Black 1** to force them to prioritize care and identify the "salvageable" patient rather than the futile patient

Yellow 1
VS on arrival: should not be done, but if the team asks, then normal

■ Summary of initial presentation: 23-year-old otherwise healthy man who was hit on the head by a small wooden board from the crash, complaining of mild headache and dizziness but denies loss of consciousness, changes in vision, neck pain, parasthesiae; is confused and otherwise stable
■ Initial interventions: patient was triaged on the scene as yellow and advised to wait in the "yellow area"
■ Physical exam
  ▶ HEENT: small abrasion on forehead, PEERL, extraocular muscles intact
  ▶ Chest: CTAB

▶ Heart: regular rate and rhythm, no m/r/g

▶ Abdomen: soft, non-tender

▶ Neuro: slightly unsteady gait but otherwise normal; alert, orientated for person/place/time, GCS 13–14

Other green/yellow patients/confederates

All green/yellow patients should be sitting quietly on the side if someone has attended to them; these patients should be consistently trickling in while the team is trying to manage patients, every 20–30 seconds, and in general will follow directions and not be disruptive.

■ Mother of dead child (**Black 1**): hysterical, crying, asking the team to save her baby; when consoled by the team, she cries quietly

■ Green 1: patient with a minor scrape on the right knee after falling from standing while running away from crash; no other injuries and a green label

■ Green 2: patient with a panic attack while witnessing the crash, no injuries and not labeled. She should be very anxious and require lots of hand holding and so on

---

Critical actions
- Termination of the resuscitation for the child **Black 1**
- Attending to mother
- Appropriate triage of yellow/green patients

Transition point 1: 2 to 4 minutes

Red 1

VS on arrival: BP 70/palp, HR 135, RR 24 94% on RA, EKG – waveform sinus tachycardia

■ Summary of initial presentation: 43-year-old patient was part of the crash with an obvious amputation (can be upper or lower extremity depending on what your center has available) but no other details are available

■ Initial interventions: EMS bandaged the amputated limb but were unable to get IV access, and they did not place c-collar; patient tagged as red

■ Physical exam

▶ General: lethargic but awake and answers questions very slowly

▶ HEENT: minor abrasion on forehead/face, PEERL, extraocular muscles intact

▶ Neck: No c-spine tenderness to palpation

▶ Chest: CTAB, no chest wall tenderness to palpation

▶ Heart: sinus tachycardia with very weak peripheral pulses and cool extremities

▶ Abdomen: minor abrasions on torso, soft, non-tender abdomen, pelvis stable

▶ Extremities: one amputation, bandaged with lots of blood seeping through; other extremities without deformities and with normal distal pulses

▶ Moves all extremities, sensation present; if the team unbandages the amputated limb, there is an arterial bleed

▶ Labs: none available

▶ Imaging: none available

Yellow 2
VS on arrival: should not be done, but if the team asks, than normal

- Summary of initial presentation: 39-year-old otherwise healthy man who fell on the right forearm while running away; patient did not hit his head and has no other injuries aside from the pain in the right forearm. He is very agitated and entitled, ripping off the yellow tag and throwing it on the floor: "I need to be seen immediately! I'm the designer of the roller-coaster, it wasn't supposed to happen! This is what you get when your production is run by the interns!" He proceeds to lie down on the free gurney if one is available
- Initial interventions: patient was triaged on the scene as yellow, given an arm sling and advised to seek medical help on his own
- Physical exam
  - HEENT: no head trauma, PEERL, extraocular muscles intact
  - Chest: CTAB
  - Heart: regular rate and rhythm, no m/r/g
  - Abdomen: soft, non-tender
  - Extremities: pain with ranging of right wrist, neurovascularly intact
  - Neuro: normal, alert, orientated for person/place/time; GCS 15

Other green/yellow patients/confederates
One or two more green patients walk in with minor abrasions.

All the greens and yellows are sitting quietly out of the way if they have been addressed, otherwise they come up to the treatment area so that they are noticed

Additional points
- If either **Yellow 1** or **Yellow 2** are placed on the second gurney, the medic complies
- If the team asks for an IV line, the medic tries but then informs the team that he is unable to obtain after several attempts; if the team does not ask for an IO, the medic can redirect them
- If the team does not tourniquet the amputated limb, the medic can redirect
- If the team asks for any other resources, EMS or the medic say that the disaster plan is activated and that the resource/transport will be here soon

---

Critical actions
- Placing the tourniquet
- IO placement and fluid resuscitation
- Complete secondary survey of **Red 1** and c-collar placement

---

Transition point 2: 4 to 6 minutes

Red 2
VS on arrival: BP 80s/50s, HR 121, RR 34 86% on NRB, EKG – sinus tachycardia

- Summary of initial presentation: 56-year-old man who was part of the crash and fell from unknown height; complaining of right femur pain and deformity, shortness of breath and right-sided chest pain. No other history available
- Initial interventions: EMS splinted right leg, placed patient on NRB; patient tagged as red

- Physical exam
  - ▶ General: older male in respiratory distress, speaking in short sentences; minor abrasion on face
  - ▶ HEENT: PERRL, extraocular muscles intact
  - ▶ Neck: no c-spine tenderness to palpation
  - ▶ Chest: abrasions and bruising to right side of chest
  - ▶ Heart: sinus tachycardia
  - ▶ Abdomen: soft, non-tender, absent bowel sounds on right, pelvis stable
  - ▶ Extremities: obvious deformity of right leg, splinted, distal pulses present; other extremities without deformities and with normal distal pulses
- If the team immediately use needle decompression for tension pneumothorax, they hear a gush of air and the patient improves: BP 116/65, HR 104, RR 24, O_2 Sat 94% on NRB, EKG – **sinus tachycardia**
- If the team focuses on the leg, if they concentrate on **Black 2** or if there is any other delay of more than 2 minutes before decompression, the patient decompensates:
  - ▶ patient is unresponsive
  - ▶ BP 85/40, HR 135, RR 42, 75% on NRB, EKG – **sinus tachycardia**
- If the team decompresses the tension pneumothorax, the patient improves; otherwise a delay of more than 1 minutes causes the patient to go into PEA arrest, which resolves only with decompression
- Team should establish IV or IO access and start 1 L normal saline

Black 2

VS on arrival: BP none, HR 0, RR agonal, no O_2 monitor, EKG – **asystole**

- Summary of initial presentation: young woman with a piece of metal stuck in the middle of her chest; EMS says she had a weak pulse in the field but has been pulseless for 7 minutes; they cannot perform chest compressions secondary to the metal in the chest
- Initial interventions: none
- Physical exam
  - ▶ General: large piece of metal stuck in the middle of her chest; no other gross deformities/signs of trauma
  - ▶ Neuro: GCS 3
  - ▶ Chest: agonal respirations
  - ▶ Heart: pulseless

Red 1

VS: BP 95/47, HR 120, RR 21, O_2 Sat 98% on NRB

- If patient continues to be fluid resuscitated, no changes in condition
- Labs: none available
- Imaging: none available

Other green/yellow patients/confederates

All green and yellow patients are cooperative.

Additional points
■ **Red 2** and **Black 2** should come in at the same time or very close to each other
■ The team needs to make one of the gurney's available for **Red 2** by moving off either **Black 2** or one of the yellows
■ If **Red 2** codes, the medic can redirect the team to consider needle decompression

Critical actions
• Needle decompression of tension pneumothorax
• Appropriate triage and reserving resources from resuscitating dead patient (**Black 2**)

Transition point 3: 7 to 8 minutes

■ Central Command should notify team that EMS units are on way and they have 1 minute to prepare the first two patients for transport; other units arriving in 10 to 15 minutes because of demand

Red 1
VS: BP 102/51, HR 118, RR 20, O_2 Sat 98% NRB

■ Changes in physical exam/patient condition: none
■ Labs: none available
■ Imaging: none available

Red 2
VS: BP 110/65, HR 104, RR 24, O_2 Sat 94% NRB

■ Changes in physical exam/patient condition: none
■ Labs: none available
■ Imaging: none available

Other green/yellow patients/confederates
Yellows/green patients should suggest that they be taken to the hospital when the ambulance arrives, but not overly distracting, except for **Yellow 2**, who is very demanding.

Additional points
■ At the 7-minute mark, there should be an EMS crew to take the first patient to the hospital
■ Team should assign one of the red patients, **Red 1**; are redirected by the medic if needed
■ 1 minute later the second ambulance crew comes for the next patient, **Red 2**

Critical actions
• Recognition of the need to transfer the sickest patient first

Transition point 4: final actions

■ Case ends when the second red patient is transferred to the hospital
■ Team should tell the other confederates that units are on way and will be taking them shortly for medical care

9. STIMULI

None.

10. BIBLIOGRAPHY

Kragh JF, Jr., Walters TJ, Baer DG, et al. Practical use of emergency tourniquets to stop bleeding in major limb trauma. *J Trauma* 2008; 64(Suppl):S38–S49; discussion S49–S50.

Timbie JW, Ringel JS, Fox DS, et al. Systematic review of strategies to manage and allocate scarce resources during mass casualty events. *Ann Emerg Med* 2013; 61:677–689.

Warner KJ, Copass MK, Bulger EM. Paramedic use of needle thoracostomy in the prehospital environment. *Prehosp Emerg Care* 2008; 12:162–168.

PART III

APPENDICES

Thinking about the cases with American Council for Graduate Medical Education milestones in mind

Lisa Jacobson

In 2012, the American Council for Graduate Medical Education and the American Board of Emergency Medicine published a joint initiative, "The Emergency Medicine Milestones Project." Twenty-three milestones were identified to help educators to evaluate the progress of trainees en route to expertise. SimWars cases provide an opportunity for program leaders to assess their residents on many of the published milestones. In addition to providing an opportunity to witness the "performance of focused history and physical examination" and "patient-centered communication," most cases also highlight the "team management skills" and "disposition skills." In addition to these four milestones, the list below identifies which cases the editors believe could be used to evaluate specific milestones.

1. Emergency stabilization (PC 1) includes those below and most others included in this text
   Case 4: Difficult airway: house fire
   Case 5: "Is there a doctor on the plane?": airplane anaphylaxis
   Case 7: Hypertensive mergency
   Case 11: Severe asthma
   Case 23: Traumatic brain injury
   Case 24: Status epilepticus
   Case 27: 27 Football injury: c-spine fracture with neurogenic shock
   Case 28: Floppy newborn resuscitation
   Case 31: Pediatric status epilepticus
   Case 32: neonatal cardiac arrest
2. Pharmacotherapy (PC 5) includes the following and others
   Case 2: Industrial fire victim: burns and cyanide toxicity
   Case 8: Adrenal insufficiency
   Case 24: Status epilepticus
   Case 26: 26 Stroke/health information technology [lytics]
   Case 34: Ondansetron and long QTc syndrome
   Case 38: Body packer
   Case 41: Migraines and beta-blocker overdose
3. Multitasking/task switching (PC 8) include
   Case 28: Floppy newborn resuscitation
   Case 29: Postmortem cesarean section with seizing neonate at delivery
   Case 33: Anaphylaxis in a patient boarding in the emergency department

Moulage in minutes

Becky Damazo

SimWars is by nature fast paced and challenging. The competition requires opposing teams to quickly assess and make diagnostic decisions. Because rapid decision making is part of the competitive arena, it is important that each team receive the same clues and be able to get a quick picture of the medical event and move forward with appropriate interventions. Moulage can help to provide clues to guide teams (Fig. B.1). It is always important to remember that the case scenario objectives and team performance is the goal of the exercise and the moulage is only one of many tools to guide participant decision making.

The problem for the moulage artist is how to create wounds and scenes rapidly and provide each team with the same diagnostic clues. There are many extensive and time-consuming moulage procedures that can be introduced into the simulation arena that are not appropriate for this setting . The following are some simple clues that can be standardized, quickly assembled and, equally important, quickly cleaned-up so that another case can be presented without interruption.

Trauma scenes are inherently covered with blood. The simulated blood products available through vendors or novelty stores can easily stain mannequins, tables and surroundings. The moulage artist should use caution when squirting blood around, with an eye to possible staining and difficult clean-up. There are a number of theatrical tricks that can be useful in the SimWars environment.

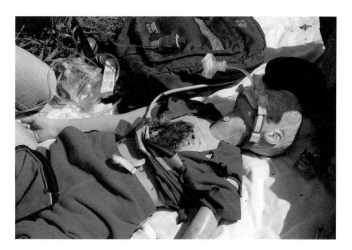

Fig. B.1
A moulage
dummy.

ADVANCED PREPARATION

When planning for the SimWars moulage, it is important to have the scenario in advance and begin to create the items needed to provide scenario realism. Do as much of the creation and staging in advance as possible.

Blood-stained items

It is convenient to prepare blood-stained bandages, sheets and clothes in a controlled location. By preparing the items in advance it is possible to have all the staged blood completely dry. This makes it easy to place blood-stained items on or around the mannequin without any fear of staining and for quick cleanup. Spritz (do not soak) lightly with a little silicone spray to create a glistening look on the surface.

Blood

Blood can be created in volume for use during scenarios. Figure B.2 shows a bottle of fake blood prepared using a combination of washable finger-paints and washing-up liquid. "Blood" can be made in advance with several bottles available to quickly add

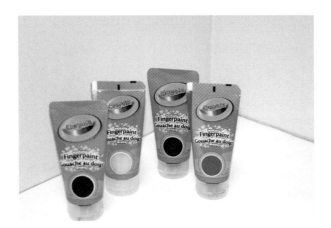
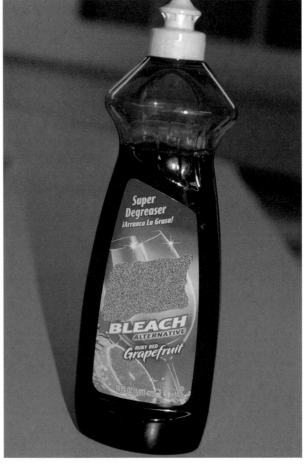

Fig. B.2 Washable finger-paints and washing-up liquid to make fake blood.

effect to the scene. It is important that mannequins be adequately protected from damage.

Barriers

The moulage artist can make sure equipment is protected and cleanup is quick by using barriers. Here are a few tips to use when placing blood or wounds on mannequins.

Think about where to place the wounds.   Mannequins typically have surfaces with varying "skin" qualities. If possible, choose the surface that is least porous for applying make-up.

Apply a barrier to the skin.   Petroleum jelly is an inexpensive and effective barrier, helpful to prevent damage to the mannequin. Just put a thin layer of petroleum jelly on to the surface of the mannequin where the wound is to be constructed. This process does two things: it provides a protective coating and it makes wound application easier; in some situations, it can replace adhesive.

If there is a lot of blood or many wounds.   Another effective barrier that is useful when there is a lot of blood or many wounds is the use of plastic wrap. Simply apply a layer of plastic wrap under the wound or involved area and it will provide a measure of protection for the mannequin.

Theatrical materials

There are a number of theatrical materials available for use with mannequins or actors that can provide an amazing level of realism.

Gel effects.   A gelatinous material can be molded into the shape of a wound and quickly applied to a mannequin. The material can be crafted to simulate wounds, rashes, blood or trauma. The use of the material requires preplanning. Figure B.3 shows a SimWars gunshot wound and blood on the bed for a trauma victim in a

(a)

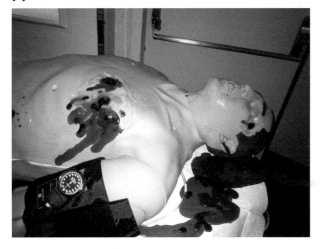

(b)

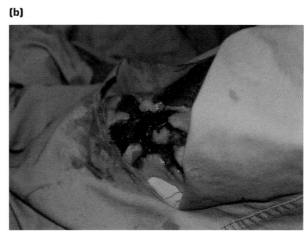

Fig. B.3 A SimWars gunshot wound (a) and blood on the bed (b).

SimWars competition. The wound cleans up in minutes and the blood peels quickly from the sheets leaving no residue. The blood in Fig. B.3a does not run but does give the visual clue needed for the competition scenario. These two items were premade and simply placed in the scene. Once the scenario is over they can be moved and stored to be reused in the next scenario. The burn at the beginning of this article (Fig. B.1) was also created using gel effects materials layered with a burn product.

Cheap (dollar store) powdered make-up.   This can be used to create bruising, bites or rashes. Bruising requires only the colors necessary to create the bruise effect, typically reds, blues, yellows and greens. These colors can be quickly applied over the petroleum barrier to create a bruise that may give clues to the patient history. In Fig. B.4 a bruise has been created to demonstrate abuse for a scenario. The rash in Fig. B.5 was created using a clear gel effects and a paintbrush with its tips dipped in powdered blush and blotted on the surface. Clean-up time for both these situations is about 10 seconds.

The gel effects material is versatile and with advanced planning can be used in a variety of scenarios. Figure B.6 shows a wound being placed that includes a glass fragment. This look was created using the same gel effects material in flesh and blood colors, with a piece of a broken plastic plate placed into the wound to create a glass impalement.

Fig. B.4 Bruise created to demonstrate abuse.

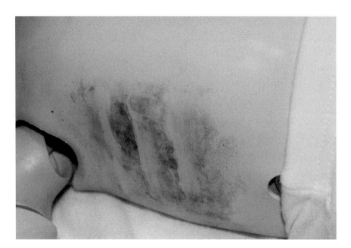

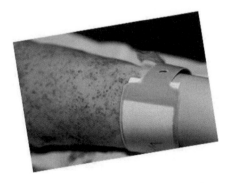

Fig. B.5 Rash created using a clear gel effects and a paintbrush with tips dipped in powdered blush and blotted on the surface.

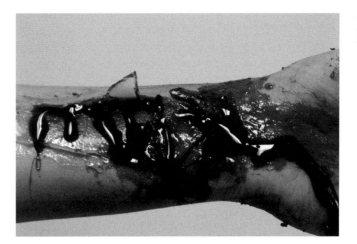

Fig. B.6 A wound with a glass fragment.

The process of designing moulage for specific SimWars scenarios should be planned to project the case clues rapidly. Like all theatrical stage make-up, the effects need to be bold and dramatic and stand out to an audience who may be viewing from a distance.

Clothes

Clothes must be easy to change for the mannequins, so cutting a slit in the back of a t-shirt or sleeve and sewing Velcro in appropriate places can make for easy clothing changes. Clothing can be burned or stained with simulated blood and dried. The clothing can be stored in plastic bags and transported to the SimWars events.

Sweat

There is anxiety in most of the scenarios and it is helpful to bring a sweat mixture (combination of glycerin and water) in a spritzer bottle to provide this clue.

Smell

Smell can be created and used to provide clues, but it is difficult to relay this sign to the audience.

Smoke

Smoke machines are helpful to create the urgency needed for fire scenarios (e.g. fire in the OR). It is important to remember that fog machines can rapidly create the smoke effect and rapidly fill an auditorium. It is then difficult to clear the air for the second scenario. It is possible to have a person manage this effect and release only enough fog to provide the clue and then use a fan to blow the smog aside during the changeover.

When planning for the SimWars moulage it is important to have the scenario in advance and begin to create the items needed to provide scenario realism. Box B.1 gives a sample packing list.

Box B.1 Sample packing list for SimWars

Gel effects wounds: two entry and two exit wounds with minimal bleeding present
Gel effects for a large pool of blood to place on gurney
Gel effects for a second pool of blood to place on floor
Bloody man's dress white shirt
Bloody sheet for gurney
Bottle of liquid blood for hands
Silicone spray
Petroleum jelly

BIBLIOGRAPHY

Alex, G. (2009) *The ATLS® Moulage – A quick guide Journal of Emergency Primary Health Care (JEPHC)*, Vol. 7, Issue 2.

Damazo, R. (2012). *Moulage and more: Theatrical tricks and amazing tools to create simulation reality*. Published at California State University, Chico. Jan. 2012.

Case images

This section contains the images to use for the cases, identified by their coded numbers.

APPENDIX C FIGURES

Radiography

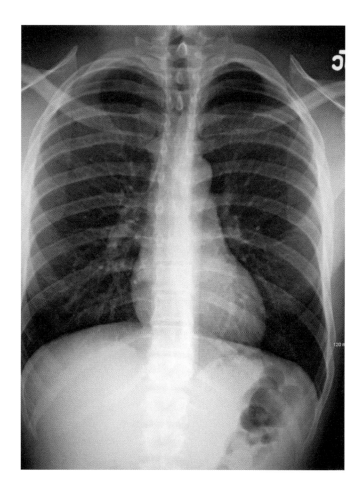

XR1 Normal male CXR. (Courtesy of Jacqueline Nemer.)

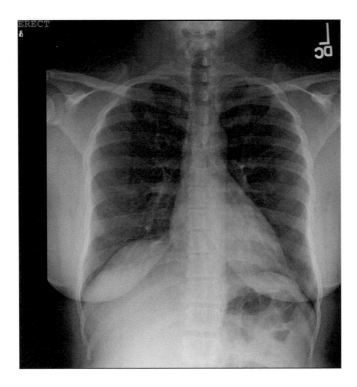

XR2 Normal female CXR.

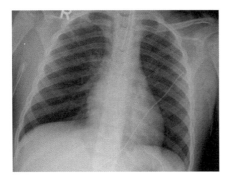

XR3 Normal male intubated CXR.

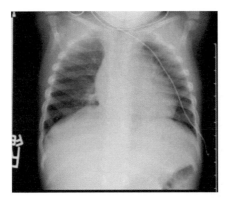

XR4 Normal infant CXR. (Courtesy of Karissa Miller.)

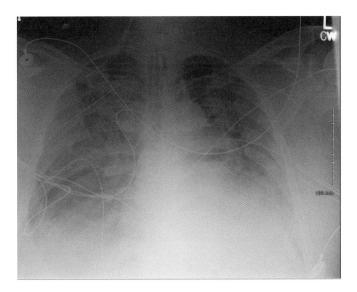

XR5 Male CXR intubated with aspiration. (Courtesy of Neal Aaron.)

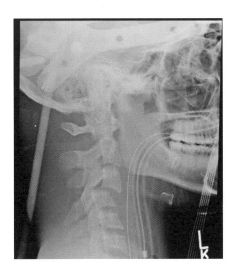

XR6 Lateral c-spine with high cervical fracture and significant intrusion on the cord.

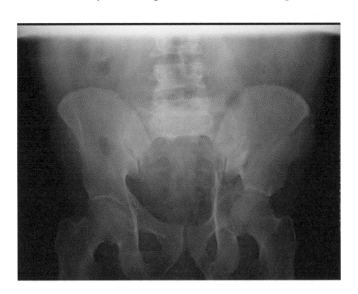

XR7 Pelvis with left acetabular fracture. (Courtesy of Paul Wasserman.)

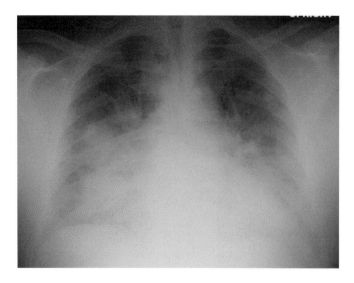

XR8 CXR with pulmonary edema.

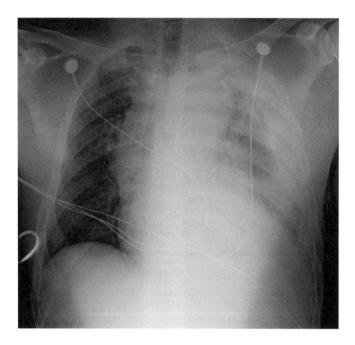

XR9 CXR with wide mediastinum. (Courtesy of Gregory Wynn.)

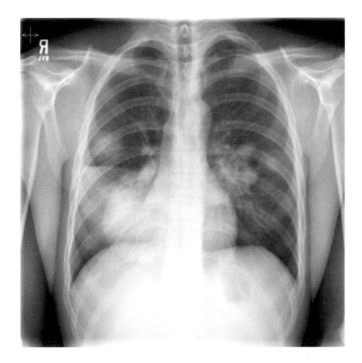

XR10 CXR with multilobar pneumonia.

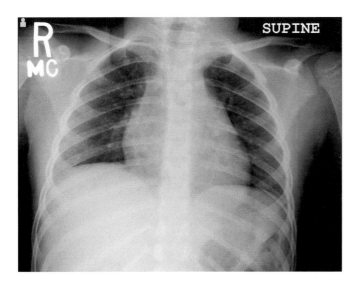

XR11 Pediatic CXR. (Courtesy of Bryant Lambe.)

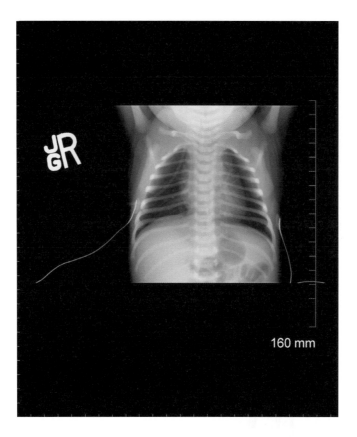

160 mm

XR12 Normal neonatal CXR. (Courtesy of Benjamin Jordan, University of Florida College of Medicine.)

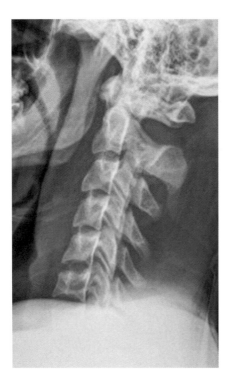

XR13 Lateral view of C1–C6, cannot visualize C7.

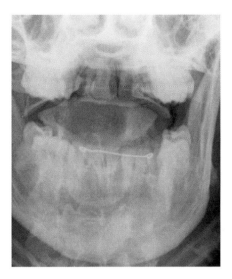

XR14 Odontoid view with C1 Jefferson fracture.

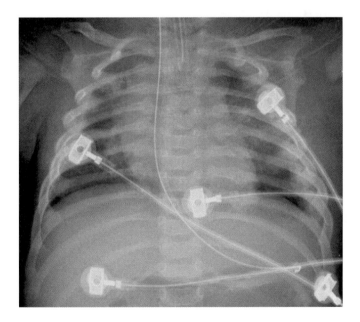

XR15 Pediatric abuse, rib fractures (intubated view). (Courtesy of Ben Hentel and radiopaedia.org.)

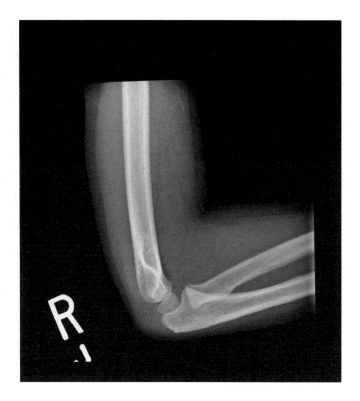

XR16 Elbow.

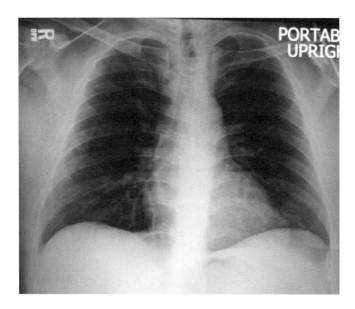

XR17 Chest.

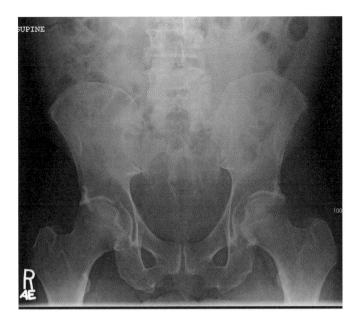

XR18 Pelvis.

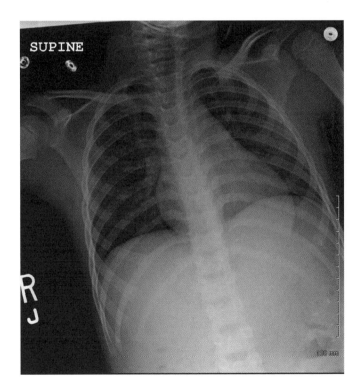

XR19 Pediatric CXR.

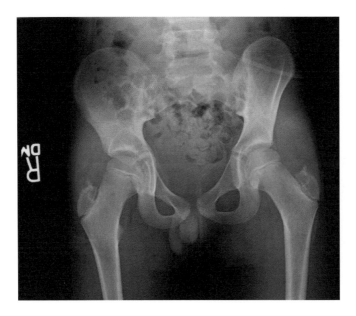

XR20 Normal pediatric pelvis.

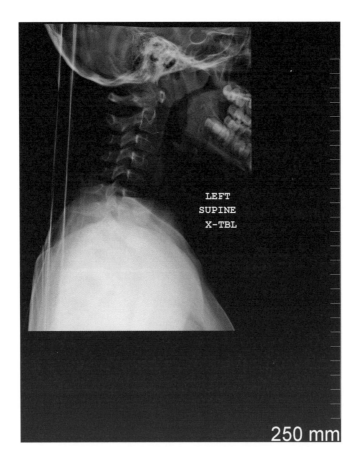

XR21 Normal pediatric c-spine (Courtesy of Benjamin Jordan, University of Florida College of Medicine.)

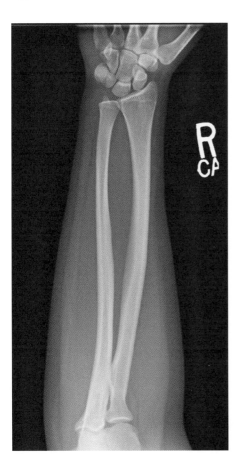

XR22 Forearm.

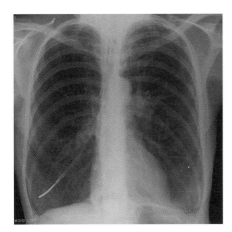

XR23 Nasogastric tube in trachea. (Courtesy of Frank Gaillard and radiopaedia.org.)

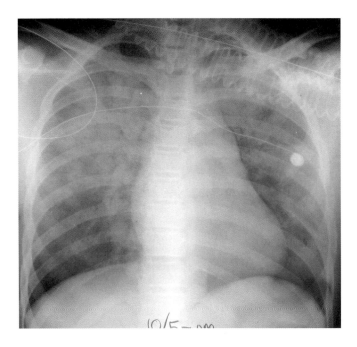

XR24 CXR with non cardiogenic pulmonary edema. (Courtesy of William Herring.)

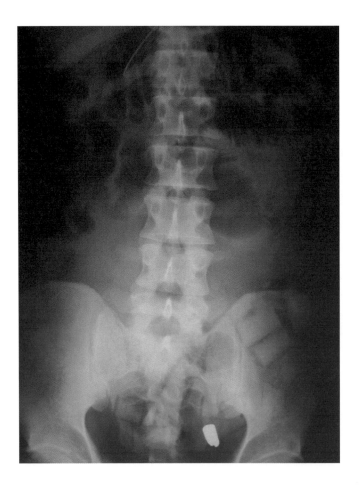

XR25 Abdomen with intestinal distention and outline of cocaine-filled condoms. (Courtesy of Gregory Wynn.)

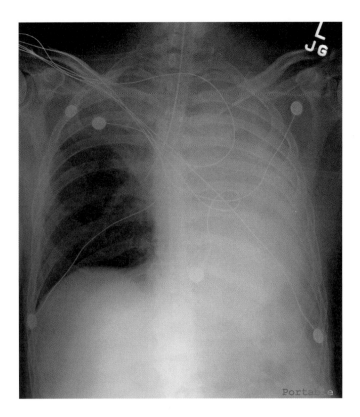

XR26 CXR with right mainstem intubation. (Courtesy of Gregory Wynn.)

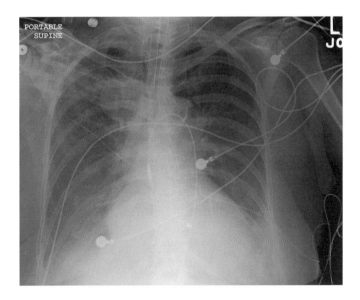

XR27 Left ventricular assist device. (Courtesy of Gregory Wynn.)

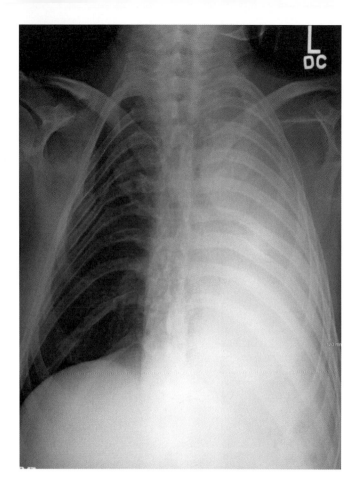

XR28 CXR with left contusion/hemorrhage/pneumothorax. (Courtesy of Kristin McKee.)

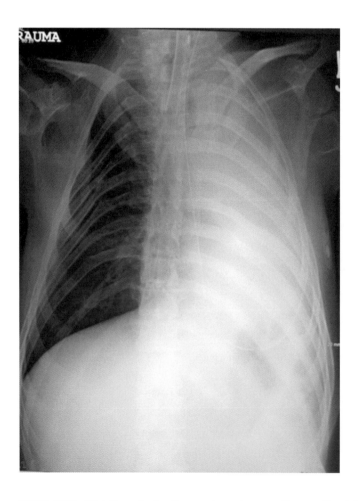

XR29 CXR with left contusion/hemorrhage/pneumothorax after intubation (Courtesy of Kristin McKee.)

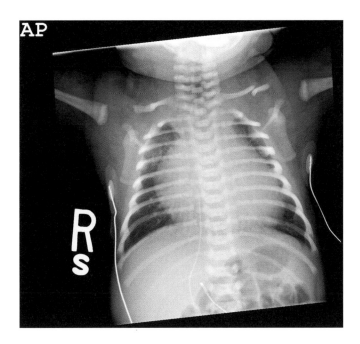

XR30 Neonatal CXR with cardiomegaly (Courtesy of Benjamin Jordan, University of Florida College of Medicine.)

Electrocardiography

Vent. rate   103 bpm
PR interval   148 ms
QRS duration   88 ms
QT/QTc   350/458 ms
P-R-T axes   49 59 38

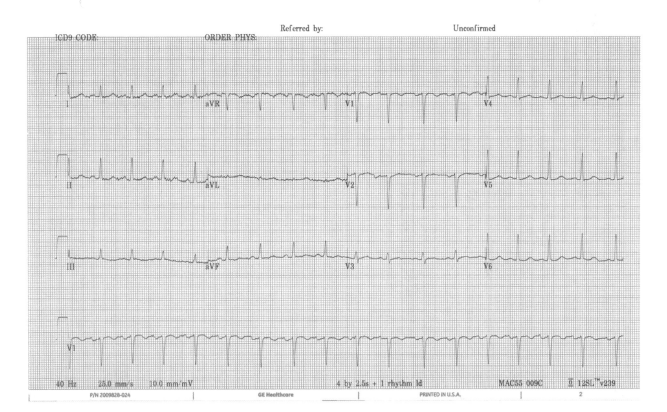

EKG1 Sinus tachycardia.

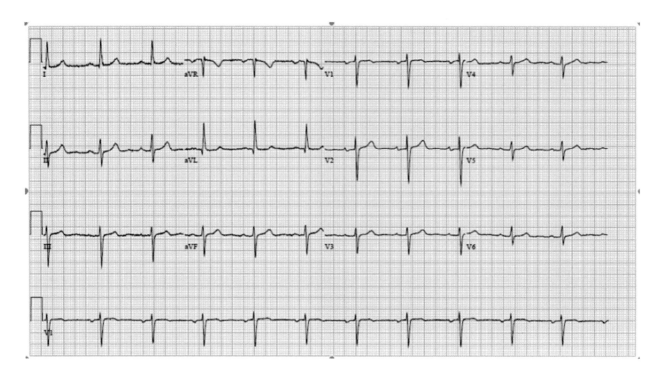

EKG2 Normal sinus rhythm.

Rate   85
PR   164
QRSD   94
QT   364
QTc   433

--AXIS--
P   69
QRS   53
T   71

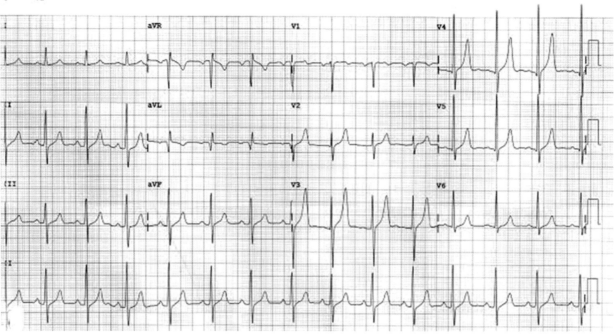

EKG3 Sinus tachycardia, normal intervals, prominent T waves.

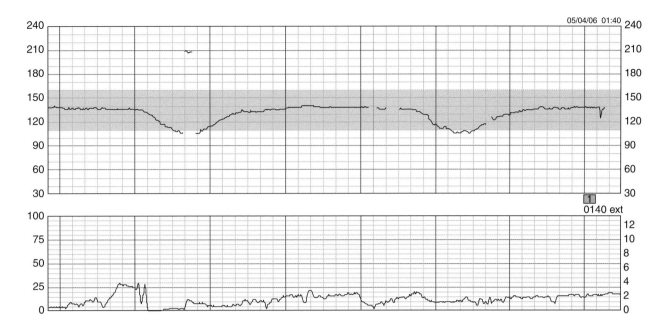

EKG4 Fetal heart.

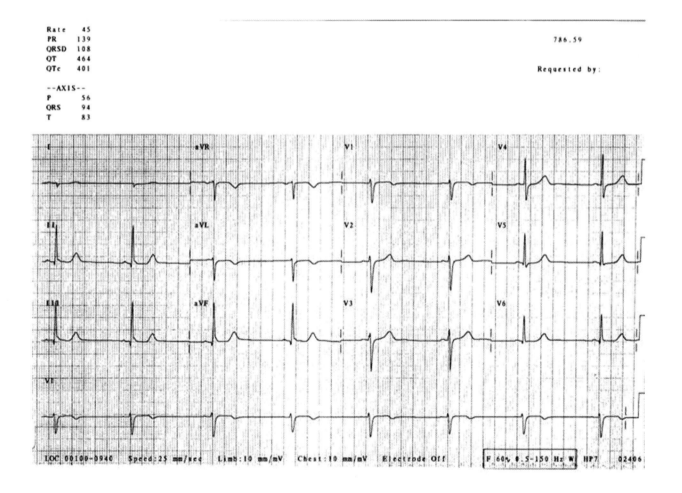

EKG5 Sinus bradycardia.

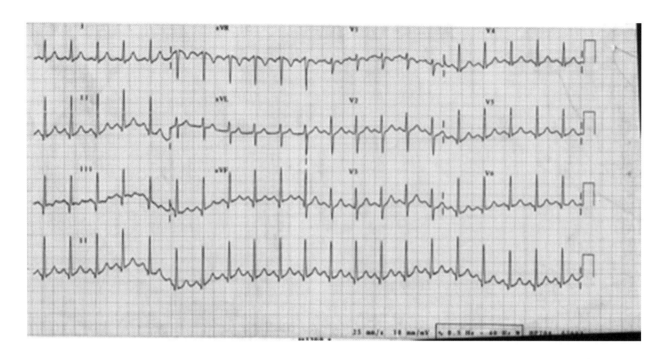

EKG6 Sinus tachycardia. (Courtesy of Jacqueline Nemer.)

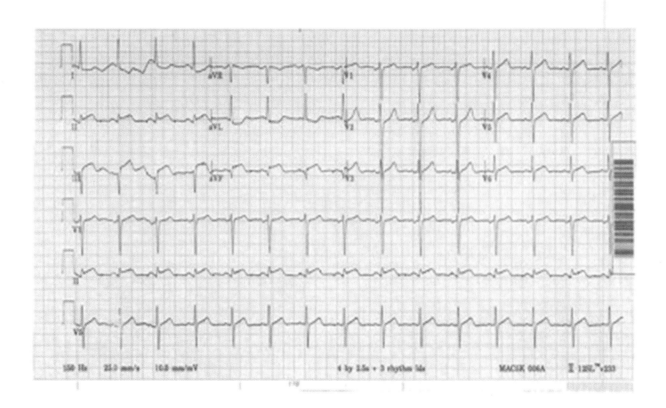

EKG7 STEMI. (Courtesy of Jason Wagner.)

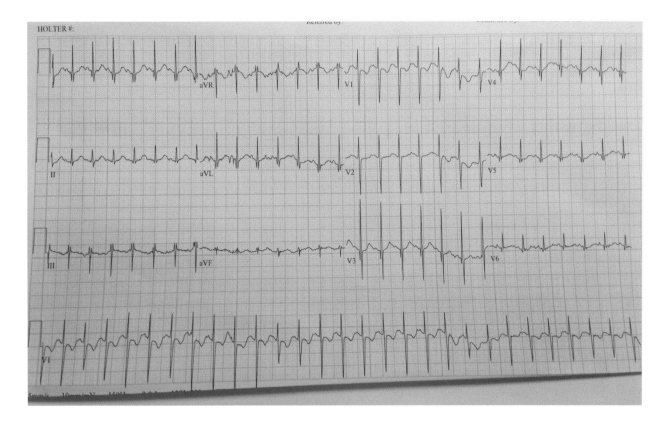

EKG8 Pediatric tachycardia.

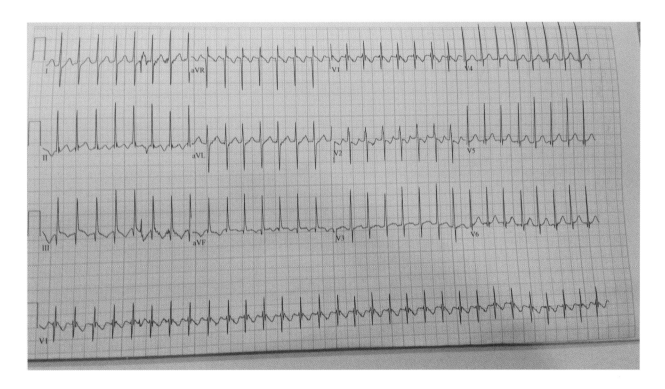

EKG9 Neonatal sinus tachycardia.

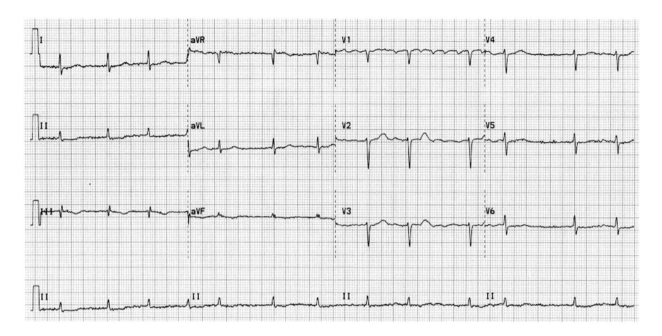

EKG10 Rate-controlled atrial fibrillation. (Courtesy of Mark Silverberg.)

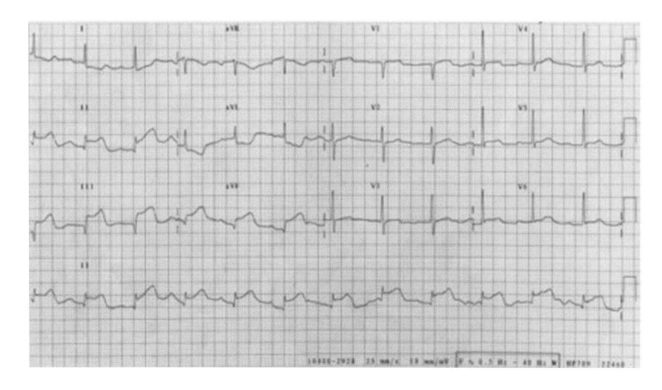

EKG11 STEMI. (Courtesy of Jason Wagner.)

Vent. rate   103 bpm
PR interval   148 ms
QRS duration   88 ms
QT/QTc   350/458 ms
P R T axes   49 59 38

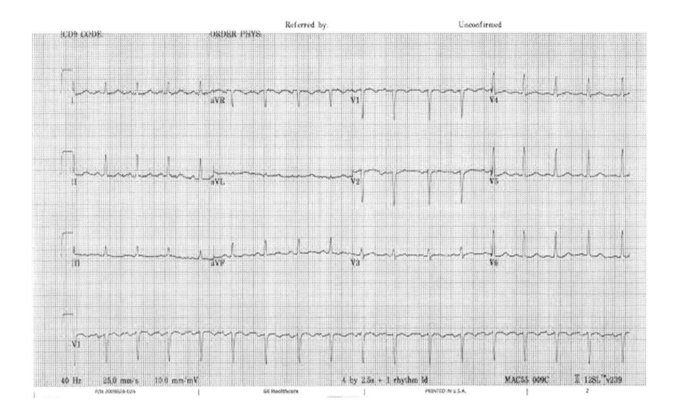

EKG12 Sinus tachycardia.

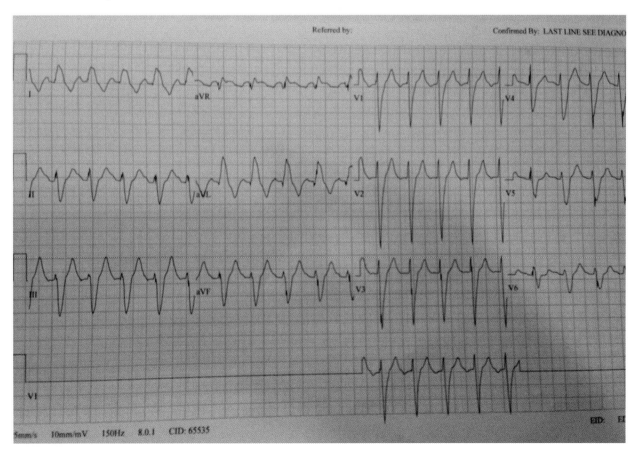

EKG13 Ventricular tachycardia.

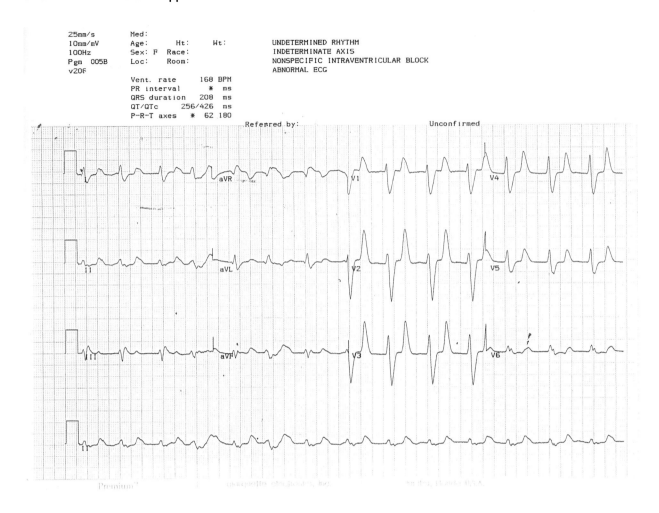

EKG14 Wide QRS. (Courtesy of Jacqueline Nemer.)

Computed tomography

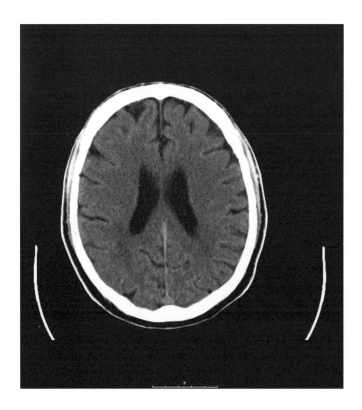

CT1 Normal head. (Courtesy of Mark Silverberg.)

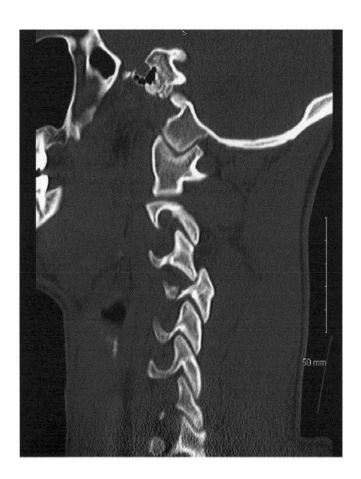

CT2 Cervical spine with high fracture. (Courtesy of Paul Wasserman.)

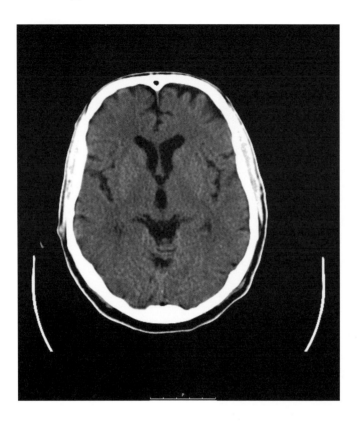

CT3 Normal head. (Courtesy of Mark Silverberg.)

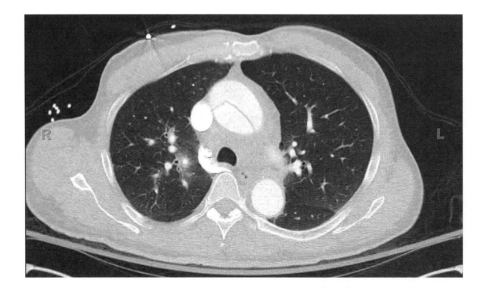

CT4 Type A aortic dissection.

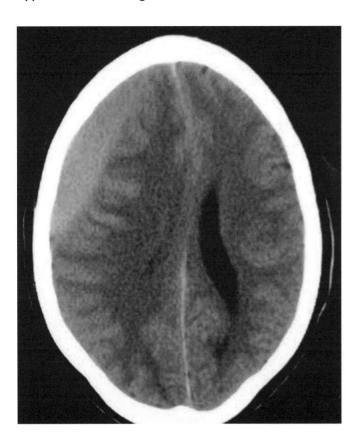

CT5 Epidural hematoma with midline shift. (Courtesy of Mark Silverberg.)

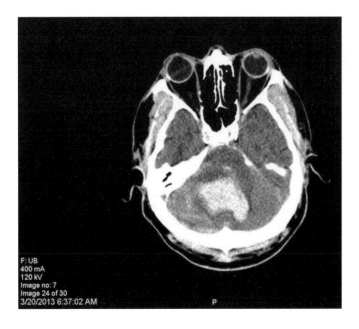

CT6 Cerebellar hemorrhage. (Courtesy of Mark Silverberg.)

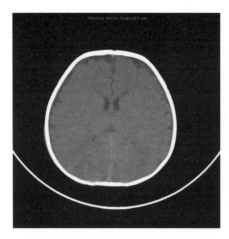

CT7 Pediatric subdural hematoma. (Courtesy of Ben Hentel and radiopaedia.org.)

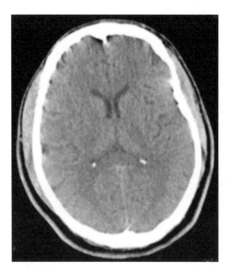

CT8 Normal head.

(a)

(b)

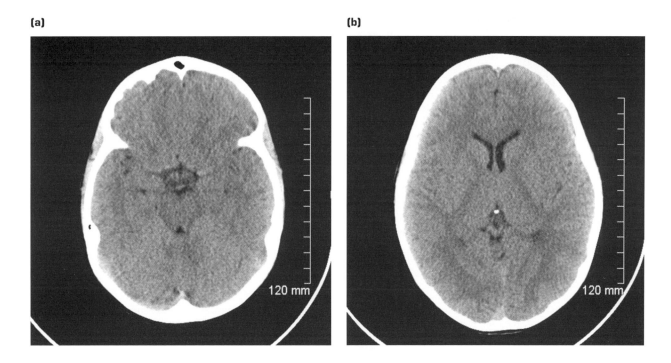

CT9 Pediatric head. (Courtesy of Benjamin Jordan, University of Florida College of Medicine.)

(a)

(b)

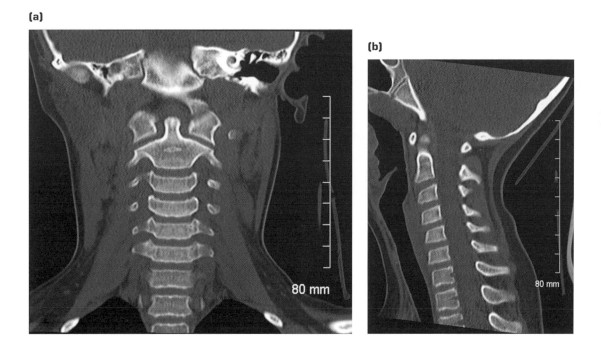

CT10 Pediatric c-spine. (Courtesy of Benjamin Jordan, University of Florida College of Medicine.)

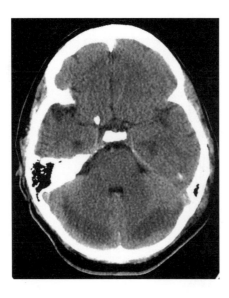

CT11 Head CT in carbon monoxide poisoning: symmetric low attenuation in cerebellum, globus pallidus and caudate nuclei. (Courtesy of William Herring.)

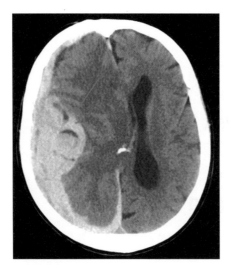

CT12 Large intracranial hemorrhage and midline shift. (Courtesy of James Heilman and Wikipedia.)

(a)

(b)

(c)

(d)

(e)

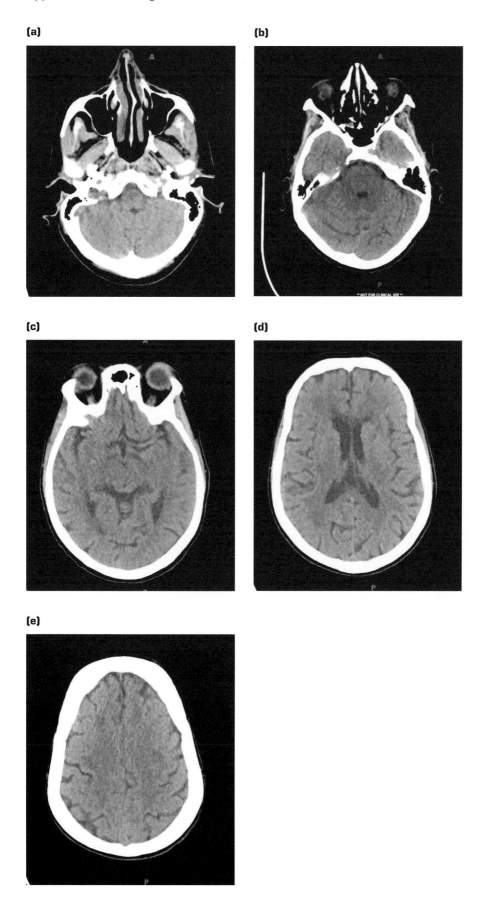

CT13 Normal head, multiple slices. (Courtesy of Jason Wagner.)

Ultrasound

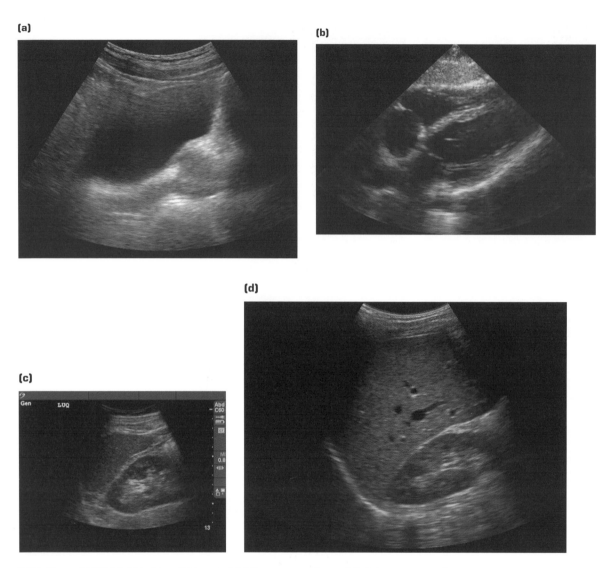

(a)

(b)

(c)

(d)

US1 Normal FAST: (a) bladder; (b) heart; (c) left upper quadrant; (d) right upper quadrant.

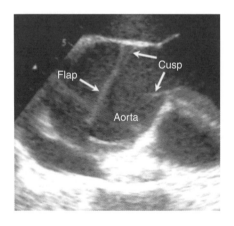

US2 Cardiac US. (Courtesy of Jason Wagner.)

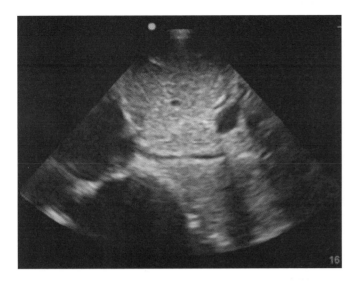

US3 Poor volume status IVC. (Courtesy of Jacqueline Nemer.)

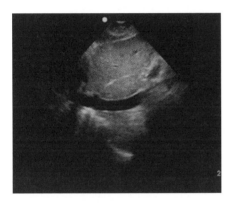

US4 Normal IVC. (Courtesy of Jacqueline Nemer.)

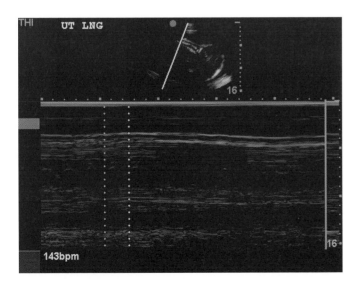

US5 Fetal heart. (Courtesy of Petra Duran.)

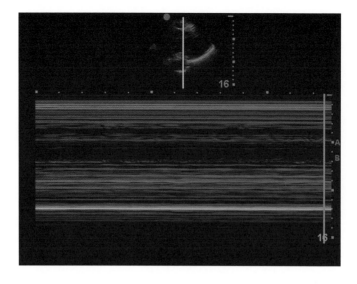

US6 female cardiac arrest. (Courtesy of Petra Duran.)

Index